31-Day

Let Jesus Love the Weight off of You

By Connie Witter, Gwen Myrie, & Sherry Riether

CONTENTS

INTRODUCTION

This is not a book about how to lose weight. Rather, this is a book about how to be intimate with the Lover of your soul. We have all read books that have given us rules to weight loss and may have even attained a small measure of success, but the results were not lasting because the root problem was not addressed.

Losing weight is a journey of the heart. The problem is not what you're eating, but what you're believing. Jesus is the only one who can guide you successfully through the tangled web of erroneous beliefs you have about yourself: lies which have been hidden deep within your heart. He is the Lover of your soul, and you will need Him to help you every step of the way!

Are you ready to have the way you think and believe about yourself transformed? Have you come to the end of your own self-effort? Are you ready to let Jesus love the weight off of you, because that is where permanent weight loss begins! The journey to weight loss is a personal one and will be tailored to your intimate needs. And, although it may seem overwhelming to you right now, you can be sure that Jesus will get you to the other side!

This book can be used as a daily devotional for your personal journey with Jesus as you let Him love the weight off of you. We have divided the devotions into a 10-week study. Consider inviting some friends to do a group Bible study together! You can use the journal pages to share with one another what you've learned and how you are applying the truth in your life.

Each week you can encourage each other to embrace your true identity in Jesus, and experience letting Jesus love the weight off of you together. It's time to live in the freedom of a healthy life that Jesus came to give us all!

The video teaching of the 10-week Bible study can be found at www.conniewitter.com.

About the Authors

Connie Witter is a speaker, author, and Bible study teacher. She is the founder of Because of Jesus Ministries, which was established in 2006. Her best-selling Bible study, *Because of Jesus*, was published in 2002 and is the foundation of her life and ministry. Her online Bible studies can be seen worldwide through her ministry website www.conniewitter.com.

Connie has traveled throughout the United States and internationally, sharing the life-changing message of *Because of Jesus*. She has been the guest speaker at churches, men and women's conferences, prison ministry, 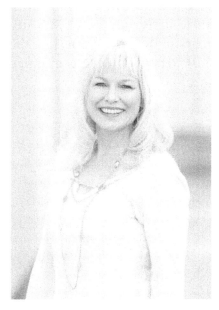 and has also spoken into the lives of teenagers. She has been a guest on several Christian TV and radio programs, and has her own nationwide weekly TV program, *Because of Jesus with Connie Witter*, which also airs in South Africa.

Connie's ministry hosts the Women of Grace Conferences that are held internationally and throughout the United States. For more information on attending a WOG conference go to: www.womenofgrace.us. If you're interested in having Connie come speak at your event, you can contact her at Connie@conniewitter.com.

Gwen Myrie

Gwen Myrie, founder of Reigning through Righteousness Ministries, is a minister of the New Covenant of grace. She is also a speaker at the Women of Grace National and international Conferences hosted by Because of Jesus Ministries. Gwen's passage out of the law and into grace came as a result of burnout from filling her life with the work of the church. Done with her self-effort to be approved by God, she cried out to Jesus to reveal Himself to her.

Now, with heart and eyes wide open, Gwen's passion is to reveal Jesus and the true heart of the Father for His children. Gwen ministers at women's conferences, Bible studies, and prison ministry outreaches. She is a graduate of Victory Bible College and Oral Roberts University's Ministry Training & Development Program. By letting Jesus love the weight off of her, Gwen has lost 50 pounds and is continuing her journey to greater health and vitality.

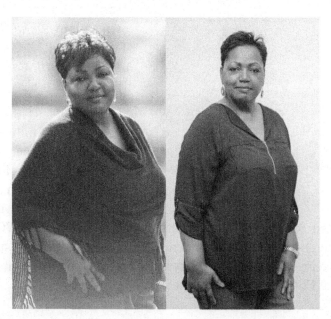

Sherry Riether

Sherry Riether co-pastors Healing Grace Church, alongside her husband, Greg. She teaches leadership classes, is a speaker at the Women of Grace Conferences and holds a full-time career as a human resource professional. As a young child, she recalls feeling surrounded by God's love, believing anything was possible. Over the years, shame, guilt, and condemnation (stemming from the belief that she was never good enough) took the place of child-like faith, and church became a place to avoid.

However, in 2007 she heard the message of grace and learned that Jesus had made her righteous and holy as a free gift. Receiving the grace of Jesus Christ has changed her life and she has stepped into her real identity as a daughter in Christ. Knowing she is completely accepted and loved, she is once again believing that with Jesus anything is possible! By letting Jesus love the weight off of her, Sherry has lost over 60 pounds and is continuing her journey to greater health and vitality.

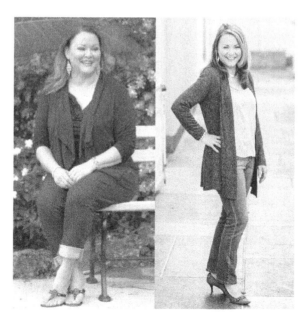

Week 1

Sherry Riether

Day 1

Let Jesus Love the Weight off of You

"2 ...What incredible joy bursts forth within us as we keep on celebrating our hope of experiencing God's glory!... 5 And this hope is not a disappointing fantasy, because we can now experience the endless love of God cascading into our hearts through the Holy Spirit who lives in us!"

– Romans 5:2, 5 TPT

Have you ever lost hope of being able to maintain a healthy weight? It's our good Father's will for all of His children to live strong and healthy lives. This is His glory for us all. Romans 5:2 & 5 tells us that this hope of experiencing God's glory in your body is not a disappointing fantasy because you can experience the endless love of God cascading over your heart through the Holy Spirit loving that weight right off of you!

Nobody ever starts out in life saying, "I'm going be fat." You just wake up one day and the pounds are on you, and they just keep piling on. It feels like you're out of control, and there's nothing you can do to stop it. I started putting on weight when I was in high school and I've struggled with weight all my adult life.

One day, I was sitting next to Gwen Myrie at a conference, and we heard Connie Witter say, "Let Jesus love the weight off of you!" Those words hit my heart. It's not that I didn't want to lose weight. I just hadn't thought of it in that context before.

3

I had really been growing in my identity in Christ. I had been speaking the truth over the circumstances in my life, but in the area of my weight it did not occur to me to speak the truth over myself. In that moment, I looked at Gwen, and she looked at me—the Holy Spirit was doing a work in both of our hearts. Since that day, it's been so fun watching both of us transform by letting Jesus love the weight off of us!

After that conference, I thought, *Well, that's funny, Jesus. I haven't thought about losing weight in a long time.* Quite honestly, at one point in my life, I had completely given up and I actually weighed 82 pounds more than I do right now. I had resigned to believing lies about myself.

I thought, *I guess I'm just meant to be fat. It runs in my family.* I had embraced the flesh identity because of what my eyes could see.

I had tried all the diet programs so many times and always failed. You can only white-knuckle it for so long, but eventually, you get sick of that soup or whatever rule-keeping system you are trying in the flesh. I'd lost hope of ever maintaining a healthy weight. The struggle was real. I felt so defeated, and I was sick of feeling defeated in this area!

Yet, after I heard the words, "Let Jesus love the weight off of you," they just kept coming back to my mind, over and over again. Then, one day I was walking through my bathroom. I looked into the mirror and said, "Jesus, if I'm ever going to lose weight, You're going to have to love it off of me, because I don't know what to do."

The change in me began to happen on another particular day when I was walking through my bathroom. I said those words again, "Jesus, if I'm ever going to lose weight, You're going to have to love the weight off of me." Right after that, I began to speak over myself, "I am at a healthy weight. Yes, I have a healthy body. I make healthy choices. I like healthy food. My skin is healthy. My organs are healthy. My mind is healthy. That's who I am."

The moment I began to speak out of my mouth what was true about me, things started to change. The hope of experiencing God's glory in this area of my life was no longer a disappointing fantasy. That day, Jesus started loving the weight off of me. He began creating in me the desire to make different choices.

As I began to embrace my true identity in Jesus, it was amazing what began to happen within me. My success did not happen when I hit my goal weight. It happened that day when I began to believe what my Heavenly Father said about me and came into agreement with Him. I was a success before I even lost one pound!

Just like Romans 5:2 says, incredible joy burst forth in me as I began to celebrate my hope of experiencing the glory of God in my body. I began to experience exactly what Romans 5:17 promises me: *"how much more will those who receive God's abundant provision of grace and the gift of righteousness reign in life through the one man, Jesus Christ!"* (NIV).

As I received God's grace, and His free gift of my righteous identity in Christ, I began to reign in this area of my life. When I look at pictures of myself during that time, I think, *Who is that person?* I have changed so much!

Letting Jesus love the weight off of you begins with asking Him to do the work within you, listening to His words of love, and speaking what He says about your body. Are you ready to let Jesus love the weight off of you? This hope of maintaining a healthy weight is not a disappointing fantasy. Jesus will love the weight off of you. It's time to receive His grace and embrace your true identity so that you can truly reign in life through Him. Let the journey begin!

Prayer: Jesus, if I'm ever going to lose weight, You're going to have to love the weight off of me. I have felt like such a failure, but I know that's not what You say about me. Today I lay my opinion of myself down, and I embrace Your opinion of me. I am a healthy weight. I make good choices. I have a healthy body. Help me to see myself the way You do. Thank You for loving the weight off of me.

Has the hope of ever maintaining a healthy weight felt like a disappointing fantasy to you? How does it make your heart feel when you hear the words, "Let Jesus love the weight off of you?" Take time to share your heart with Jesus. Let Him love you today!

_____

_____

_____

_____

_____

_____

_____

_____

_____

_____

_____

_____

_____

_____

_____

_____

_____

_____

_____

_____

_____

_____

_____

Day 2

Come to the Throne of Grace

"So now we come freely and boldly to where love is enthroned, to receive mercy's kiss and discover the grace we urgently need to strengthen us in our time of weakness."

– Hebrews 4:16 TPT

I cannot tell you how many times I have said to myself, "This time, I'm serious. I will lose weight!" Then out came the list: go to the gym and exercise, avoid overeating, reduce calorie intake, "give up" soda, or chocolate, or chips, or pasta, or...

I even tried doing one of those programs through my work where the nurse would call me and send me emails about healthy living. "Weight management" they called it! Ha! I "managed" to find all kinds of ways to avoid talking to that person on the phone and ended up deleting the emails. Why? Why couldn't I stick with something and see it through to the end? Or, if I was successful and lost weight, why did I always regain it all, plus more? Why didn't I just have more self-control?!

Often, obesity is not a self-control issue. It's a heart issue. This issue of the heart has its roots in an overwhelming sense of lack that silently shouts the lie inside our minds that we are worthless, there is something wrong with us and then demands, "Do something about it!"

Our hearts are desperately searching for something we can do to silence the accusing voice of lack and find healing. That's when we try in our own self-effort—in our "flesh"—to heal our own hearts. When we try to find healing on our own, we will only be successful for as long as our flesh-strength holds out. Someone once said, "Anything that is begun in the flesh, must be maintained in the flesh."

How much better is it if there is an inner strength that comes from grace, a grace that flows into and through a heart that is complete in Christ? Healing for your heart only happens from the inside—when we receive and experience God's unconditional love and acceptance. This is what allows our hearts to find healing. Grace is defined as "The Divine influence upon the heart, and its reflection in life."[i]

When we turn to Jesus and take our hearts to Him, we find grace. He's the Lover of our souls. Do you believe that? Do you believe that He loves and accepts you right now, and that you are complete in Him right now? To receive that is to enter into the influence of grace.

Let's read Hebrews 4:16 again, *"So now we come freely and boldly to where love is enthroned, to receive mercy's kiss and discover the grace we urgently need to strengthen us in our time of weakness"* (TPT).

To "receive mercy" means to find help for our weaknesses. The answer to our weaknesses is found in His grace! He wants us to receive his "Divine influence upon our hearts" when our hearts are showing forth neediness. The healing of our hearts by His acceptance and love is the key to overcoming weaknesses. We can come boldly to Him! "Boldly" in this verse means "with unreserved speech."[ii]

Basically, it means getting real with Jesus! He knows your heart, anyway, so why not let it out? Tell Him what you are feeling, how hard it is, and even tell Him what you're angry about. The reality is, your struggle with food likely began as something completely different than a simple desire to eat.

As you bring your heart to Him, He is going to immediately begin to bathe your heart in love and acceptance. "There is nothing wrong with you. You are all fair, my love. You are lovable and perfect to me because you are complete in Christ." It is within those whispers of love from Song of Solomon 4:7, Hebrews 10:14, and Colossians 2:10 that you will find the beginning of your journey to health. You are not alone in this! You can come to the throne of grace!

When I finally came to the end of my self-efforts with weight loss and getting healthy, I told Jesus, "If I am ever going to lose weight, it's up to you!" I came to Him with this! And He took me at my word. I believe that when I said those words to Jesus, He began working in my heart at that very moment. Through the journey, He would bring many things into my life to get me to my end goal, but the most important of these was to help me see myself differently.

I began agreeing with what He says over me. I am complete in Jesus. I have everything I need to be healed, whole and healthy. I told Jesus, "I'm going to believe what You say, that You love and accept me."

Come boldly to Him right now! Come to the throne of His grace, His influence of love and acceptance upon your heart. Believe me, you will find the help that you need. Healing begins right now.

Prayer: Jesus, I thank You that I can boldly come to You and bare my heart to You, and You will meet me right where I am with grace and tender mercy. I thank You that as I let you begin to heal my heart, You are always on my side, in my corner, cheering me on. Thank you, Jesus, for Your great love for me that leads me to make good choices and empowers me to know I have self-control and that I am a success. I know You will love the weight off of me.

What thoughts and desires would you share with your very best friend and confidant; someone you completely trust? Share those with Jesus! That's what it means to boldly approach the throne of grace with confidence. Let Jesus begin to heal your heart from the inside out.

Day 3

Not My Willpower but His Real Power

"[Not in your own strength] for it is God Who is all the while effectually at work in you [energizing and creating in you the power and desire], both to will and to work for His good pleasure and satisfaction and delight."

– Philippians 2:13 AMPC

I tried to get healthy and lose weight repeatedly, but it never worked. In my own flesh, my abilities, I couldn't do it. I would diet and lose weight, but it would come right back and more pounds with it. Dieting just felt like defeat to me, and I didn't need one more failure: one more area where I just couldn't do it—where I didn't have any strength to do it.

At one point, I finally decided that being at a healthy weight was impossible for me. I said to myself, "Obesity runs in my family. I'm a big girl and I'm just going to be a big girl because that's what I'm meant to be." I started embracing that false identity, which ended in utter defeat and I just gave up.

Some may say that giving up is resting in Jesus. I disagree. Do you know what giving up got me? Giving up got me to 222 pounds! Giving up is not the answer. Giving up means to resign yourself to failure, and that failure only brought me more guilt, more shame, and more defeat. God did not create us to fail! That's not "resting in Jesus."

However, there truly is a rest to be found, and it's in God's power that is at work in us. Philippians 2:13 says that it's God's power that is creating in us the desire and ability to accomplish His good pleasure, satisfaction and delight. So, what is His good pleasure and satisfaction and delight? It's that we come into our identity as His children.

His good pleasure is that we embrace the identity in Christ given to us as a free gift. What is that identity? Our identity is that we are complete in Him and we lack nothing! When we received Jesus as our Savior, He came to live on the inside of us and brought everything that He is with Him. Is Jesus unhealthy? No! Does Jesus struggle with food addiction? No! Does Jesus have self-control? Yes!

Whatever is true about Jesus is true about you because you are one with Him! 1 John 4:17 says, *"As He is, so are we in this world"* (NKJV). Declare this truth over yourself today: "As Jesus is, so am I in this world!"

When I began to see that receiving my identity in Christ needed to be applied in every area of my life, including my health, I started coming into agreement with what my Heavenly Father says about me. I began to declare the truth to myself and say, "I am healthy. I am at a healthy weight. I make healthy choices. I like healthy food. I don't have to eat that whole bag of potato chips. I can pass on the Double Tree cookies they brought into work today."

When I would say these things, it would cause faith to rise in me and manifest in strength to make a healthy choice. That's when things began to change. The next thing I knew, my diet soda habit that had held control over me for more than 10 years just fell right off of me! With no self-effort!

I didn't try to break that habit. It wasn't even a goal! Yet, one day I realized that I wasn't craving it and I didn't need it anymore. This was a significant breakthrough for me! You have to realize that for more than 10 years, I always had to have a diet soda in my hand. I drank it all day! When I realized that habit was gone, I knew Jesus was working in me to change me!

You see, it was not my willpower, but His real power that was at work in me! His real power was energizing me and creating in me the ability and desire to keep going toward my goal of being healthy. Realizing that it's Jesus' power, His work and His strength at work in me has made the difference. It helped me make changes to my eating habits and even inspired me to exercise.

His desire and His energy came alive within me. It created in me the desire and the ability to make different choices. Relying on His strength and power led me to begin resting in Him regarding my weight and my health. When I began to rest, Jesus showed me what would work for me to lose the weight. Rest in His real power and He will show you what will work for you. He will lead you on your own individual path.

Prayer: Jesus, I thank You that I don't have to rely on my own strength to lose weight and get healthy. I agree that it is Your power that is alive in me, because You are alive in me. Your power is creating in me the desire and the ability to make healthy choices. I know You are working in me now because You love me. Thank you, Jesus, for helping me to agree with what You say over me. I am complete in You. I am healthy. I make healthy choices. I can do all of these things in Your strength. Amen.

Say this out loud: "Father, I receive Your identity. I boldly confess that I am Your child and I lack nothing! Your Spirit is alive in me and I know it's Your power at work in me, energizing and creating in me the ability and desire to be healthy." Meditate on these words and capture the thoughts Jesus is speaking to your heart.

_____

_____

_____

_____

_____

_____

_____

_____

_____

_____

_____

_____

_____

_____

_____

_____

_____

_____

_____

_____

_____

Week 2

Gwen Myrie

Day 4: Help Me, Jesus!

Day 5: You're Tall and Slim Like a Palm Tree

Day 6: It's a Heart Issue

Day 4

Help Me Jesus!

"Listen carefully, my dear child, to everything that I teach you, and pay attention to all that I have to say.
21 Fill your thoughts with my words until they penetrate deep into your spirit.
22 Then, as you unwrap my words, they will impart true life and radiant health into the very core of your being.
23 So above all, guard the affections of your heart, for they affect all that you are. Pay attention to the welfare of your innermost being, for from there flows the wellspring of life."

– Proverbs 4:20-23 TPT

I remember the day that "Help Me Jesus!" became the cry of my heart. I had hit rock bottom. I weighed 237 pounds and was as miserable as can be. There was nowhere to go. I was defeated, depressed and condemned! I had tried so many times to lose weight and failed every time. I knew that I could not do this on my own, in my own strength. Not until I realized that my self-effort was not going to cut it, did I let go and cry out: "Help Me Jesus! If You don't persuade my heart that I can change, I will die fat."

That was the beginning of me asking Jesus to love the weight off of me. I knew that Jesus was going to rescue me from this bondage and persuade my heart of His truth about this area of my life!

How does Jesus rescue us? Psalms 107:20 tells us: *"He sends forth His word and heals them and rescues them from the pit and destruction"* (AMP).

God will always send His Word to you. You may not be aware of all the times He does this, but you can be sure that He does. Have you had a friend speak a word to you? Have you listened to a message at church? Or have you opened your Bible and a verse popped out to you? These are the many ways God sends His Word to rescue you. Take the time to recognize all the ways that your good Father sends His Word to you. You'll be amazed at how many times He does!

Proverbs 4:20 says, *"My son, attend to my words"* (KJV). What does it mean to "attend" to God's Word? God's Word is what He believes and knows is the only truth about you. Jesus said in John 17:17, *"Sanctify them by your truth. Your word is truth"* (NKJV).

The word "attend" means "to hear, to pay attention, and give attention to." [iii] We know that Jesus is the Word of God made flesh, so this Scripture is saying, "Pay attention to what Jesus is saying to you and about you or give Jesus your attention." The Truth is speaking, and He wants you to give your attention to Him. He will only speak the truth about who you are. He can be trusted for He will never lie to you!

When our good Father sends forth His Word to rescue us, we all have the choice to either believe it or reject it. What we choose to do with God's Word will determine the course of our lives.

I want to share something that happened to me at a conference I attended in Chicago, IL. I was listening to my friend, Connie Witter, minister the Gospel from a passage in the Song of Songs. The Bridegroom was speaking to the bride telling her how beautiful she is to Him, but she responded by rejecting what He said about her. With every word of affirmation that the Bridegroom would speak over the bride, she would discard what He was saying.

While Connie was speaking, the Holy Spirit, who is the Spirit of Truth, began to minister to my heart with these words. "Did you ever hear the stars say to Me, 'We aren't coming out tonight,' or the sun say, 'I don't think I will shine today?' In other words, all of creation knows and obeys My voice except my highest creation—man."

In Genesis, when God speaks, we see that He is creating. When He speaks, He is calling those things that be not as though they are. He told me that day to agree with Him when He calls me beautiful. In that moment I said, "Yes, Lord, I am beautiful. I agree with what You say about me." God was not telling me I was beautiful in order for me to become beautiful. He was speaking over me what was already true about me because God cannot lie!

That day was a turning point in my life because I began to embrace what He was saying to me. That day I gave attention to His word of truth, and His Word began to determine the course of my life. That was the day Jesus began loving the weight off of me.

In Proverbs 4:21-22, your good Father encourages you to fill your thoughts with His words until they penetrate deep into your spirit. Then as you unwrap all that He says about you, His words will impart true life and radiant health into the very core of your being.

Prayer: Jesus, thank you for always sending your Word to rescue me. I will pay attention to what you say about me. Your Word brings true life to me and radiant health to the very core of my being. I choose to believe what You say about me.

You have the power to either believe or reject what Jesus says about you. What did He speak to your heart in today's devotion? How will you respond to His words of life?

Day 5

You're Tall and Slim Like a Palm Tree

"Oh, how delightful you are; how pleasant, O love, for utter delight! 7 You are tall and slim like a palm tree..."

– Song of Songs 7:6-7 TLB

Jesus' definition of slim and the world's definition of slim are two different things. Our Jesus sees us at a healthy weight. When He looks at you, He sees His righteous, victorious, glorious bride. You are so delightful to Him. He sees you flourishing like a palm tree (Psalm 92:12). When it comes to your body, He sees you as just right in Him!

Growing up I took on a false identity. I did not see myself the way Jesus saw me. Instead, I embraced what the world said about me. I was called "Fatso" as a kid, and I embraced that as my identity. So, for the better part of my childhood into my adulthood, I struggled with my weight.

What I've come to discover is that our heart belief is the location of the core issue. We live from our hearts. The identity that I believed about myself was that I was a fat person. I believed that losing weight was hard because I had done the Dr. Atkins diet. I had done the Mediterranean diet. I had done a grapefruit and cabbage diet. I tried everything to lose weight, every rule keeping system. I could be successful for a little while through my own self-effort, but the weight always came back, plus its buddies.

I eventually came to the end of myself, the end of my self-effort. I was attending Connie Witter's Bible study and she made this statement: "You are tall and thin like a palm tree! That's what Jesus says about you!"

I thought, *Well, that might be what Jesus says*, but I wasn't buying it. I thought, *Is this woman really looking at me? Or is she just trying to be nice?* On another occasion, when I was at Bible study, I recall her quoting Psalm 92:12: *"The righteous shall flourish like a palm tree..."* (NKJV).

In the Passion Translation, Psalm 92:12 says, *"Yes! Look how you've made all your lovers to flourish like palm trees, each one growing in victory, standing with strength!"*

When I heard this truth, I decided to look up the characteristics of a palm tree. I discovered that one of the characteristics of a palm tree is that it sheds dead weight. That really hit me. I thought, *If I flourish like a palm tree, then that's what's true about me. I shed dead weight.* In that moment, Hebrews 12:1-2 came to my mind. These verses say to lay aside every sin and the weight that so easily besets us, and we do this by keeping our eyes on Jesus, the author and finisher of our faith.

I realized that it was the sin of unbelief that had beset me. I had not been believing what Jesus said about my identity, and that's what was weighing me down and holding me in bondage to a constant struggle with my weight. But the answer was to set my eyes on Jesus, the author and finisher of my faith.

When that Scripture came to me, I said, "Yes, Lord, persuade my heart of this truth." We have to understand that weight loss is a heart issue. It's an identity issue. What do we really believe about ourselves? Who am I? If the belief of your heart doesn't change, you'll stay trapped in a case of mistaken identity.

So, the Lord began to unravel the wrong beliefs in my heart about my identity. He said to me one time, "Gwen, there is no condemnation for those who are in Christ Jesus" (Romans 8:1). See, I had been walking around with the sense of being condemned because I had done all these diets and failed, but when He said that, I could feel the freedom coming into my heart.

I remember at one of the Women of Grace Conferences that Sherry Riether and I attended together, Connie Witter made the statement, "Jesus is going to love the weight off of you!" I thought, "That's right!" That was another one of those words of persuasion and the nickel finally dropped. My heart was persuaded that I could be changed by His love.

Jesus has done this work in my heart, and I've lost over 50 pounds! It was the easiest 50 pounds I have ever lost because of the simple fact that I stopped trying and embraced my true identity in Jesus.

A lot of people have asked me, "Gwen, how did you lose all your weight?" I'm very reluctant to tell them what I did because I don't want them to follow a specific set of rules and be unsuccessful, once again. So, what I tell them is, "Sit your butt down, and let Jesus persuade your heart about your true identity. You're tall and slim like a palm tree. That's right! You shed dead weight! You're righteous in Jesus, and you flourish like a palm tree!" That's what's true about you! Let Jesus persuade you of who you are. Let God change the way you think about yourself, and He will love the weight off of you.

Prayer: Jesus, help me to see myself the way You do! If You say I'm tall and slim like a palm tree, then that's what's true about me! I receive your love today by agreeing with what You say about me! I shed dead weight and flourish like a palm tree because I am righteous in You! Your love sets me free!

Read Song of Songs 7:6-7 again. How does it make your heart feel to hear Jesus say these words to you? No matter what you see in the mirror, Jesus sees you as healthy and victorious. You are the delight of His heart. Will you let Jesus love you today by embracing what He sees when He looks at you?

_____

_____

_____

_____

_____

_____

_____

_____

_____

_____

_____

_____

_____

_____

_____

_____

_____

_____

_____

_____

_____

_____

_____

Day 6

It's a Heart Issue

"Keep and guard your heart with all vigilance and above all that you guard, for out of it flow the springs of life."

– Proverbs 4:23 AMPC

Can it really be that simple? Do we really live from our hearts? Proverbs 4:23 says above all, guard your heart, for out of it flow the springs of life. What we believe is so powerful that it shapes our very lives. Proverbs 23:7 tells us that as a man thinks in his heart, so is he. You are living in the results of what you have believed in your heart about yourself.

Romans 10:10 says, "For with the heart a person believes..." (AMPC). This is a powerful Scripture because it shows you where belief begins. All our problems and struggles come from the beliefs of our heart. It is crucial that we know that our hearts are the issue because, until then, we will constantly search for solutions elsewhere. I want to talk to you about the importance of believing the truth about yourself because we live from our hearts, and the Scripture bears this out.

Proverbs 4:23 says, *"Guard your heart above all else, for it determines the course of your life"* (NLT). Did you catch that? There are things that we believe about ourselves, whether lies or the truth, that will determine the course of our lives.

We are just like our Father God. He believes and then He speaks. The Scripture says that out of the abundance of our hearts, our mouths speak.

Luke 6:45 says, *"A good man out of the good treasure of his heart brings forth good...for out of the abundance of the heart his mouth speaks"* (NKJV).

When God made man, He made us in His image, His likeness. The way we create is just like our Heavenly Father. We believe and then we speak.

2 Corinthians 4:13 says, *"And since we have the same spirit of faith, according to what is written, 'I believed and therefore I spoke,' we also believe and therefore speak"* (NKJV).

I would like to emphasize that what we believe in our hearts is what we speak from our mouths. And what we believe in our hearts is what will manifest in our world. Let's look at this principle as it worked negatively in my life.

Practically all my life I believed that I was fat and unlovable. These were prevailing thoughts and beliefs that shaped my life. And I had plenty of reinforcements of this belief. I heard it from my family, kids at school, and when it was time to buy clothes. For the better part of my life, I struggled with trying to lose weight and gaining it all back because I did not address the issue residing in my heart.

Defeat was my constant companion. I lived in inner turmoil because I believed that my life would never change. Needless to say, my outer world manifested what I believed in my heart. Insecurities, loneliness, and isolating myself from people was the fruit of my life. When I did go around people, I pretended that I was happy with who I was, but on the inside my world was spinning out of control. What I believed in my heart was manifesting in my life.

Although this truth can have negative results, this is actually a good thing because the moment we embrace what God says about us, it will change our inner world, which will begin to reflect in our outer world. In other words, when we believe the truth about ourselves, that will also manifest in our lives!

Our good Father has given us a good heart and has put a new spirit in us. That old way of believing died at the cross of Jesus Christ. Colossians 2:14 says, *"...Everything we once were in Adam has been placed onto his cross and nailed permanently there as a public display of cancellation"* (TPT). Now we are equipped to believe good things about ourselves with our good hearts.

You might ask, "How do I know my heart is good?"

Ezekiel 36:26 says, *"And I will give you a new heart—I will give you new and right desires—and put a new spirit within you. I will take out your stony hearts of sin and give you new hearts of love"* (TLB). God has fulfilled this promise in the New Covenant through our Lord Jesus Christ. We can boldly declare, "I have a new heart!"

Look again at Luke 6:45: "A good man out of the good treasure of his heart brings forth good..." (NKJV).

Because God says that you are good, and He has given you a good heart, you can plant in your good heart the things that Jesus says about you. His desire is for you to embrace every word that He says so that you will experience good fruit in your life. It is time to manifest who you really are by believing and speaking what Jesus says about you.

Prayer: Father, thank You for showing me the importance of guarding my heart. By the power of Your grace, I will only believe and speak what You say about me. You have given me a good heart that believes the truth. I live by every word that You say about me, and I will see Your Word manifest in my life. Thank You for showing me the truth that sets me free!

Did you know that what you believe in your heart will manifest in your life? How does it make you feel to know that Jesus has given you a good heart? Take time today to speak what Jesus says about you out of the good treasure of your heart.

Week 3

Connie Witter

Day 7

The Struggle is Over! You Have the Mind of Christ!

"...But we have the mind of Christ...and do hold the thoughts (feelings and purposes) of His heart."

– 1 Corinthians 2:16 AMPC

I've been growing in grace and my identity in Christ for a long time, but one day I found myself struggling with negative thoughts. I know that I'm the righteousness of God in Christ, and I began to speak what God said is true, but for some reason I couldn't get rid of the fearful thoughts that were bombarding my mind. The struggle was real, and I felt like I was drowning underneath these oppressive thoughts.

Jesus has brought me to a place where my heart is consistently at peace, so this experience was foreign to me. I normally feel very confident about what my good Father says about me, so I didn't understand what was happening. I finally asked Him, "Father, what is happening to me? Why can't I get victory over these negative thoughts? Show me the truth that will set me free!"

In that moment, He spoke to my heart and revealed to me something about my identity that set me free. One hundred percent of the time when we're struggling in an area of our lives, it's a case of mistaken identity. We're believing something about ourselves that isn't true.

I knew I needed a fresh revelation of who I am in Christ. That is the only place I've ever found true, lasting peace and joy. So that day, as I listened to the Holy Spirit within me, I heard, "Connie, you have the mind of Christ. Embrace your true identity concerning your thoughts and your mind."

Immediately, 1 Corinthians 2:16 came into my thoughts. I had never really thought of the mind of Christ as part of my righteous identity. I had quoted that Scripture and believed it, but this was a much deeper revelation the Holy Spirit was giving me. It was a revelation about my identity concerning my mind and my thoughts that would change my life forever!

Let's read 1 Corinthians 2:16 again: *"...We have the mind of Christ...and do hold the thoughts (feelings and purposes) of His heart"* (AMPC).

As I thought upon this verse, the word "have" jumped out at me. The mind of Christ was not something I was trying to get. This Scripture said I have it!

This word "have" means "to own it; to possess; to lay hold of." [iv]

That meant I own the mind of Christ! I lay hold of His thoughts, feelings and purposes of His heart as my true identity. WOW! A light bulb came on that day. The Holy Spirit revealed to me that Jesus had already won this struggle I was having by giving me His very mind.

The word "struggle" means "to make strenuous efforts in the face of difficulties or opposition; struggling with a problem; to proceed with difficulty or with great effort." [v]

Every struggle in our lives, including the struggle to lose weight and get healthy, is in our minds. The way we are thinking and believing is determining our failure or success. Trying to believe right and do right by our own self-effort causes us to struggle. Jesus came to deliver us from our self-effort. He said, *"Keep company with me and you'll learn to live freely and lightly"* (Matthew 11:28-30 MSG).

That day when I came to Jesus, He taught me how to live freely and lightly by reminding me who I am in Him. When I let go of my self-effort and owned the mind of Christ as my true identity, the struggle was over! Embracing identity is a very powerful, spiritual thing that changes everything in a person's life.

The world says, "The Struggle is Real! You need to try harder to overcome this battle with your weight. You need to exert strenuous effort to think right and do right so you can be healthy." That's self-effort!

Jesus says, "The Struggle is Over! I overcame this battle for you! I gave you My mind! You can let go of your strenuous self-effort to lose weight and let Me do the work in you." That's grace!

Every struggle begins in your mind. What you think about yourself determines the very course of your life. Proverbs 4:23 says, *"Be careful how you think; your life is shaped by your thoughts"* (GNT). The health of your body is shaped by your thoughts! That's how imperative it is that you embrace the truth that you have the mind of Christ so you can live a long, healthy life.

How you think about food is shaping your life. A thought comes into your mind before you put one bite of food in your mouth. Those thoughts control the way you eat, how much you eat, and what you eat. The good news is you don't have to be controlled by unhealthy thoughts about food anymore. You can let the Holy Spirit change the way you think by embracing your true identity in Jesus.

You hold the thoughts, feelings, and purposes of God's heart about food. As Jesus is, so are you in this world. So, the next time you find yourself struggling with a negative thought about food, you can boldly say, "The struggle is over! I have the mind of Christ!" Jesus will work in you and create in you the desire and power to live a healthy lifestyle as you trust Him to do the work within you.

Prayer: Father, today I own the mind of Christ as my true identity. I hold Your thoughts, feelings and the purposes of Your heart toward myself concerning my health and my eating habits. I surrender my self-effort, and I trust You to change the way I think so I can enjoy Your will for me and live a long, healthy life. Thank You for loving this weight off of me!

Take time today to talk to Jesus about the struggle you have had with your weight. Are you ready to surrender your self-effort and embrace your true identity in Him? Can you see how embracing the mind of Christ as your identity has the power to change this area of your life?

_____

_____

_____

_____

_____

_____

_____

_____

_____

_____

_____

_____

_____

_____

_____

_____

_____

_____

_____

_____

_____

_____

_____

_____

_____

_____

_____

_____

Day 8

Let God Change the Way You Think

"Stop imitating the ideals and opinions of the culture around you, but be inwardly transformed by the Holy Spirit through a total reformation of how you think. This will empower you to discern God's will as you live a beautiful life, satisfying and perfect in his eyes."

– Romans 12:2 TPT

When we let the Holy Spirit transform the way we think, we live beautiful lives. Our souls are satisfied in the truth that, in Christ, we are perfect in our Father's eyes. If you've been in church very long, you've heard messages on renewing your mind. It's so important that your mind is renewed, but you must realize this isn't something you must do on your own. It's a work of God's Spirit within you. When you understand that it is God who changes the way you think, you can simply rest and embrace God's grace to help you think right.

Romans 8:6 says, *"Now the mind of the flesh [which is sense and reason without the Holy Spirit] is death... But the mind of the [Holy] Spirit is life and [soul] peace [both now and forever]"* (AMPC).

This verse describes two different ways to live. Reasoning without the Holy Spirit produces death in a person's soul; but inviting the Holy Spirit into our thoughts produces life and peace. Jesus sent the Holy Spirit to be your comforter, helper, strengthener, and to guide you into all truth (John 14:26). He sent Him to help you think right and bring peace to your mind and heart.

James 4:5-6 says, *"Or do you suppose that the Scripture is speaking to no purpose that says, The Spirit Whom He has caused to dwell in us yearns over us and He yearns for the Spirit [to be welcome] with a jealous love?* ⁶ *But He gives us more and more grace (power of the Holy Spirit, to meet this evil tendency and all others fully). That is why He says, God sets Himself against the proud and haughty, but gives grace [continually] to the lowly (those who are humble enough to receive it)"* (AMPC).

What a powerful Scripture! It says the Spirit of God yearns within us to be welcome with a jealous love. When you are struggling in an area of your life, He longs for you to ask Him to help you. Maintaining a healthy weight is an area in which many of God's children struggle.

Have you ever felt frustrated with yourself because you can't seem to eat right and exercise so that you can live a healthy life? Have you ever struggled with your thoughts about food? This is the time to ask Jesus to help you change the way you think. Embrace the truth that you have the mind of Christ when it comes to food and receive His grace to empower you to live free in this area of your life. God gives His grace to those who are humble enough to receive it.

Philippians 2:13 says, *"[Not in your own strength] for it is God Who is all the while effectually at work in you [energizing and creating in you the power and desire], both to will and to work for His good pleasure and satisfaction and delight"* (AMPC).

48

Philippians 2:13 totally changed my life. My mind used to be filled with negative thoughts about myself. Thoughts of fear, doubt, and shame brought death to my soul. I lived my life reasoning without the Holy Spirit for many years. However, I remember the day when the Holy Spirit revealed to me that I didn't have to struggle in my own strength anymore. Instead, He would create in me the desire and power to carry out God's purpose for my life.

I began to pray this verse over myself. I simply asked Him to strengthen and empower me. I found myself effortlessly thinking differently, believing differently and seeing myself differently. I didn't realize it at the time, but the Holy Spirit was changing the way I thought, and I began experiencing the mind of Christ by the power of the Spirit.

As I embraced my true identity in Christ, my thoughts began to change. I began to feel confident, secure, and loved! I began to think about myself differently and I wasn't struggling anymore in my thoughts. One day I asked the Father, "Why does it seem so easy for me to believe what You say, and yet I see so many of my brothers and sisters in Christ struggling to believe you?"

The Spirit of God said to me so clearly that day, "Connie, it's because you continue to ask me to create in you the power and desire to do what pleases Me. You asked Me to help you, you embraced what I say about you, and I have empowered you to believe Me!" I was in awe that day as I realized that the Gospel was so simple.

Yet so many Christians are still struggling in their own effort to think right and believe right when the Holy Spirit is within them, just waiting for them to ask for His help and embrace what He says about them!

If you've been struggling in your mind with depression, guilt, shame, or discouragement in the area of your weight, look to Jesus and embrace the truth that you have been given His very mind as a gift of His grace. Trust Him to change the way you think, and you'll find your thoughts changing effortlessly by the power of the Holy Spirit! You'll begin to experience the beautiful life that Jesus came to give you!

Prayer: Heavenly Father, thank You for sending the Holy Spirit to comfort, encourage, and strengthen me. Today I look to You and ask the Holy Spirit to change the way I think about food so that I can experience the healthy life that Jesus came to give me.

Take time today to talk to Jesus about how you think about food. Invite the Holy Spirit to change the way you think in this area of your life. Let Jesus love you today!

Day 9

Negative Thoughts are Not Your Thoughts

"Be careful how you think; your life is shaped by your thoughts."

– Proverbs 4:23 GNT

Thoughts are powerful! Scientists have confirmed that negative thoughts create stress which upsets the bodies hormone balance, depletes the brain of chemicals required for happiness, and damages the immune system. Negative thoughts are toxic. Scientists tell us that 87-95% of current mental and physical illnesses come from our thought life.

The affect that thoughts have on your mind and body are a matter of life or death. Your life is shaped by your thoughts. Every word you speak, every decision you make, and every action you take begins in your thoughts. This is why embracing the truth that the mind of Christ is your true identity is imperative to your entire well-being. This truth has the power to end the struggle you have had with your weight and bring health to your body!

1 Corinthians 2:16 says, *"...We have the mind of Christ... and do hold the thoughts (feelings and purposes) of His heart"* (AMPC).

You have the mind of Christ, and the mind of Christ doesn't think negatively about you. Jesus gave you His mind. His mind is filled with love, joy, peace, and self-control. Any thought that does not produce the fruit of the Spirit in us is not our thought!

Since you have the mind of Christ, this means that every negative thought that enters your mind is not yours! It didn't originate from you. So where do these negative, destructive thoughts come from?

1 Peter 5:8 says, *"Stay alert! Watch out for your great enemy, the devil. He prowls around like a roaring lion, looking for someone to devour"* (NLT).

Since scientists have proven that negative thoughts actually have the power to bring destruction to our minds and our bodies. Negative thoughts are obviously what the devil uses to destroy our health and our lives. It's imperative that you understand that negative thoughts are not your thoughts so that you'll be equipped to guard your heart from every negative, toxic thought that enters your mind.

2 Corinthians 11:3 says, *"...I'm afraid that just as Eve was deceived by the serpent's clever lies, your thoughts may be corrupted and you may lose your single-hearted devotion and pure love for Christ"* (TPT).

God spoke to Eve and said, "You are just like Me! You are good, so very good, and I approve of you completely. You are excellent in every way!" (Genesis 1:27, 31).

That was the mind of Christ toward Eve! In that moment, she experienced the very life of God. The Bible says her heart was free from all fear and shame. Then the devil came to corrupt her mind with his lies. Negative thoughts about herself filled her mind. These thoughts were not her thoughts. They did not originate from her. They came from the voice of death, the enemy of her soul. They were toxic and their purpose was to produce death in her.

Eve embraced those negative thoughts as her own and believed the lies of her enemy. As a result, her heart, which was once filled with the life of God, was now filled with fear and shame which brought death to her soul.

The exact same thing is still happening in the thoughts of God's children today. The apostle Paul said, "I fear that just like the devil corrupted Eve's thoughts with his lies, he would do the same thing to you" (2 Corinthians 11:3). Jesus gave you His righteous identity. He gave you His righteous mind, so any negative thought that tries to enter your mind is not your thought. It's the enemy corrupting your thoughts with his lies.

Since I've embraced this powerful truth that negative thoughts are not my thoughts, I've become very aware of any negative thought that enters my mind. When the voice of death tries to corrupt my mind with a negative thought about myself, I simply say, "Not today devil! That thought is not my thought, and I refuse to embrace it! I have the mind of Christ!"

If someone offered me poison, I would not drink it! That's how I see negative thoughts. They're toxic to the life of God in me. They're designed by the enemy of my soul to destroy my life and I refuse to drink his poison!

When you understand that negative thoughts are not your thoughts, you won't take ownership of them. They'll lose their power to condemn you or make you feel guilty.

Romans 8:1 says, *"So now the case is closed. There remains no accusing voice of condemnation against those who are joined in life-union with Jesus..."* (TPT).

The Case is Closed! The struggle is over! You have the mind of Christ! Any negative thought is the accusing voice of condemnation. Romans 8:1 says there remains no more accusing voice of condemnation against you because you are one with Jesus! You have His mind!

Negative thoughts come at us all, but if you believe that the negative thoughts that enter your mind come from you, they'll have the power to condemn you your whole life, and keep you trapped in the struggle to lose weight. But when you understand this powerful truth, you won't tolerate negative, condemning thoughts in your mind anymore. When a negative thought comes at you, you'll respond, "Not today devil! That's not my thought! I have the mind of Christ!" The negative, toxic, accusing thoughts of the devil will have lost their power to condemn you, and you'll truly begin to reign in this area of your life!

Prayer: Father, thank You for revealing to me today that negative, accusing thoughts are not my thoughts. They have lost the power to condemn me. I can see the struggle to lose weight has been in my thoughts, but now I know I have the mind of Christ. I trust You to help me think right in this area of my life. Thank You for loving me!

How does knowing that negative thoughts are not your thoughts empower you to resist every condemning thought about your weight? Take time today to talk to Jesus about this.

_____

_____

_____

_____

_____

_____

_____

_____

_____

_____

_____

_____

_____

_____

_____

_____

_____

_____

_____

_____

_____

_____

_____

_____

_____

_____

_____

_____

_____

_____

_____

Week 4

Sherry Riether

Day 10

Recognize the Lies That Have Held You Captive

"Then we cried out, "Lord, help us! Rescue us!" And he did! 14 His light broke through the darkness and he led us out in freedom from death's dark shadow and snapped every one of our chains."

– Psalm 107:13-14 TPT

Have you ever had that moment when you failed big time? I certainly have. When it's happened, my first reaction used to be to wallow in self-berating dialogue, feeling like I needed to spend some time experiencing self-punishment. I knew that feeling was a lie, but this had happened to me so many times that it was hard for me to stop believing that lie about myself.

One particular time stands out to me. Not long ago, I blew it one morning. I yelled at the kids. I mean really yelled at them, and I felt so horrible about it! I thought, *These poor children! This is the way they get to start their day!* While driving to work, I could hardly think of anything else. Tears were streaming down my face as the lies came to my mind: "Look what you did! You broke their hearts. You're a terrible parent! They are always going to remember how horrible you were to them!"

When I arrived at work, I sat in the dark parking garage replaying the situation in my mind and believing the lies about what a terrible parent I was. These thoughts plagued me, and it seemed like I couldn't escape them.

As I sat there, the morning sun broke through the window and it was so bright it could not be ignored. At first, I was annoyed with the light! I thought, *I'm sitting here having a pity-party for myself, believing the lies that I'm a horrible person, and now here this bright sunshine is streaming through into this dark garage!*

I turned my head this way and that way, but no matter which way I turned, I couldn't get away from the bright sunlight. Finally, I just leaned my head back against the seat of my car and gave up trying to get away from the light.

Then something funny happened. The light, that once seemed so intrusive and annoying, was suddenly warm and inviting. I began to relax and let the warm sunshine bathe my face. The next thing I knew, I wasn't upset or sad any longer. In fact, I started laughing! With the relentless sunshine streaming in, I could no longer sit in the darkness and believe lies about myself.

The sunshine that streamed in through the window so brightly that I couldn't ignore it or get away from it reminded me of the relentless love of the Father. He will not leave us in darkness, even if we seem to want to stay there. That morning, the light of His love enveloped my heart and disrupted the darkness! That's when I felt Him speak to my heart. He said, "The moment you fail is exactly the moment you should come to Me! Yes, that was a mistake, but there's nothing you and I can't do together." Suddenly, life flooded my soul and I got out of that dark parking garage with a spring in my step and new hope for the day!

This word is one that I have returned to multiple times on my journey to a healthy weight. Times when I have overeaten and felt like giving up or when I let lies deceive me. After I achieved my weight loss goal, I found that I had put a few pounds back on, and I began to experience some self-condemning thoughts again: "You'll struggle with your weight all of your life. Obesity runs in your family. Just get used to it—you're going to be on a diet the rest of your life! You can't keep the weight off! Who do you think you are, speaking and writing about 'Let Jesus Love the Weight Off of You?'"

Lies! Lies! Lies! This is when the light of God's love faithfully disrupts the darkness and I feel the warmth of His love as I remember His words to me, "There's nothing you and I can't do together!" The lies, just like the darkness, cannot stick around in the light of His love.

Jesus said, *"...I am the light of the world. Whoever follows me will never live in darkness. They will have the light that gives life"* (John 8:12 ERV)

Whoever follows Him will never live in darkness! Why? Because darkness is nothing! Do you know what darkness is? It's merely the absence of light! That's it! All I do is turn to Jesus and let his love light destroy the darkness and fill me with His life!

You might be saying, "Sherry, I have these thoughts, too, and I can't seem to get rid of them! When I fail, when I blow my diet, how do I focus on Jesus and to get rid of the self-condemning thoughts?"

First of all, you don't. You don't get rid of anything. Jesus does! Let Jesus cleanse your mind with His Word. Ephesians 5:26 says that we are bride of Christ. He gave up

His life for us to make us holy and clean, washed by the cleansing of God's Word. Jesus does it! Just listen to His words over you!

Ephesians 5:27 says, *"He did this to present her to himself as a glorious church without a spot or wrinkle or any other blemish. Instead, she will be holy and without fault"* (NLT).

Jesus made you holy and without fault! Listen to what He says over you and let Him love those lies right out of you!

Prayer: Thank You, Jesus that Your love is my light and my life! Darkness cannot, and does not, have any power! I am holy and without fault because I am Your bride. You did it! I didn't make myself Your bride. You declared that I am Your bride and You presented me to Yourself, perfect. Thank You, Jesus, for reminding me of the truth that brings me new hope!

Take some time to reflect on being the bride of Christ. Embrace and enjoy the light of Jesus' love and experience the warmth and peace He brings. Listen to His words in your heart and capture them below to remind you of the truth that you are holy and without fault.

Day 11

Let Jesus Love You Out of Your Secrets

"But I have trusted and relied on and been confident in Your lovingkindness and faithfulness..."

– Psalm 13:5 AMP

If you are someone struggling with an addiction—whether it's drugs, alcohol, or food—you don't want anyone to know. But going it alone rarely works. Why do you think so many programs out there encourage you, or even require you, to have an accountability partner, someone you must be responsible to during your program? This can be good and does help some people find success. But sometimes what was meant to be encouraging begins to feel like chastisement and condemnation when we make wrong choices.

When you fall short, fail completely, or you just don't want to do it anymore, you tend to start avoiding the person who was supposed to be helping you. Usually it is either because you have failed in your goals—or because you secretly just want to eat that candy bar and you don't want to hear, "You really shouldn't eat that."

I used to play this game of "Hide and Eat." I would hide my binge eating by doing it when no one was around. I would make an errand to the store, buy that candy bar, eat it in the car, and then stuff the wrapper in my pocket to throw away later. I was trying to make myself not feel as badly about making a wrong decision by deceiving others.

But, really, who was I deceiving? I was practicing self-deception and living a life of secrets and hiding. Someone once said, "You're only as sick as your secrets." This is true. When you are battling something, keeping it to yourself—keeping it a secret—is a road to destruction.

There is a downward spiral in self-deception. If we keep it to ourselves, shame and self-condemnation can take over and we will find ourselves repeating the same mistakes. What is the solution? The solution is life on God's terms: living life in the light!

Colossians 1:13-14 says, *"God rescued us from dead-end alleys and dark dungeons. He's set us up in the kingdom of the Son he loves so much, the Son who got us out of the pit we were in, got rid of the sins we were doomed to keep repeating"* (MSG).

Jesus brings everything into the light of truth. And guess what? It's perfectly safe there! There is no hint of condemnation from Him. His light is a place of full acceptance and love. He's not ashamed of you! He's not even disappointed in you!

Can I tell you a truth about disappointment? For Christ-followers who are in love with Jesus, we project a sense of disappointment on Jesus when we fail. It comes from our love for Him. We love Jesus and we feel badly when we fail because we feel that we have disappointed the Lover of our souls. But Jesus is never disappointed in you!

Disappointment requires unmet expectations. For Him to be disappointed would mean that you didn't meet His expectations of you. But Jesus knows us thoroughly. He knows every decision we will ever make. It's impossible for Him to be disappointed in you because He sees you as you really are—as Himself! How can He be disappointed when He sees you as Himself? He's not disappointed in Himself, so He's not disappointed in you! Don't buy into the lie of God's disappointment over your failures. That will only lead to more shame. Your failures do not define you!

Jesus' only desire is for us to be lifted back into the place of light and truth. He wants you to experience His complete love and acceptance. That's the place where shame is dead! That's the place where condemnation is dead. It's the place of new beginnings. It's the place of new strength; the strength to break old patterns.

If you fall, just run to the light of His love. That is where you will find a truly fresh start. When I began to let Jesus shine the light of His love on my heart, my downward spiral of self-deception ended. I quit trying to hide things and opened up to the One who loves me in the middle of my struggles and defeats. There is power in this!

Romans 8:1-2 says, *"With the arrival of Jesus, the Messiah, that fateful dilemma is resolved. Those who enter into Christ's being-here-for-us no longer have to live under a continuous, low-lying black cloud. A new power is in operation. The Spirit of life in Christ, like a strong wind, has magnificently cleared the air, freeing you from a fated lifetime of brutal tyranny at the hands of sin and death"* (MSG).

You no longer have to live under that continuous, low-lying black cloud! A new power is in operation. The Spirt of life in Christ is in you! He's there for you and He will never depart. When you are confident in the One who loves you, you can confidently confide in Him. Here is your freedom!

Prayer: Jesus, how wonderful You are! Thank You that You are never disappointed with me or ashamed of me. I will remember today to abide in Your love. I know I can trust in, rely on, and be confident in Your loving kindness and faithfulness to me. Thank You for loving me out of my secrets.

You can trust Jesus! He will never condemn you or be disappointed in you. He has given you a new power to live in! It's a power that sets you free from repeated mistakes. As you abide in His love, write down the empowering thoughts He is whispering to your heart today.

Day 12

Your Exodus—Let Jesus Lead You Out

"For those who are led by the Spirit of God are the children of God."

– Romans 8:14 NIV

"All of these devotionals are great, but how do I lose the weight? Do I follow the Keto diet? Do I drink shakes? Do I reduce my calorie intake? What do I do?!" By now, you may be asking these questions and may be experiencing some frustration.

This book of devotions has been going after weight loss in a completely different way. That's because the root of all unhealthy habits are matters of the heart: the thought patterns generated by wrong belief.

"But Sherry, no one can lose weight for me. I'm the one that has to do it and I need to know how!" On one hand, you are correct. If you have struggled with your weight like I have, continuing to do the same things you've done in the past will not get you to your goal of being healthy.

However, as a believer, you have Jesus on the inside of you, so you can do it with Him! And Guess what? He is your best coach, your biggest cheerleader and most loyal fan! He will be there encouraging you, helping you and convincing you of your identity in Him.

You can believe you can lose the weight and God is so good, He will reveal to your heart the right plan for you. He gave you the mind of Christ so you have the knowledge of what to do that will work this time! He will reveal your own path to you.

All through the scripture we see examples where God told His people to go and do something when they didn't have all the details of how it would be accomplished. He told Abraham to leave the only place he had known and go to the land He would show him. There was a promise of a better life, but Abraham didn't have all the details. God was showing him and guiding him as he took each step. The point is—Abraham started down a path.

We know what and how much we eat matters and that exercise is good for us. How about starting down the path by just making one change?

Not sure which one thing to do? Ask Jesus! I guarantee you, as you meditate on Him and ask Him for help, your thoughts will drift to one thing that you have peace about that will not seem so overwhelming or hard to do.

I remember when Jesus led me to drink more water. Water is a natural appetite suppressant and it is so good for you! In fact, before I began my journey, I had heard that when we think we feel hungry we are actually experiencing thirst. I read an article in a medical journal that stated that feelings of hunger and thirst ride a very thin line and are often mistaken.

I found this to be true. When I felt hungry, I would drink a full glass of water. Then if I still experienced hunger after several minutes, I would eat something. This is an example of one choice, one decision I made that helped me. I found that what and how much I ate was very much influenced by how much water intake I had for the day. These little things began to add up and they prepared me for larger changes in my eating patterns.

Everyone has an idea of the best way to lose weight, but the truth is only Jesus truly knows what will work for you. You are led by God's Spirit. All you have to do is ask Him, and He'll show you an individual path that will be effective!

When I didn't know what to do, I said, "Jesus, if I'm ever going to lose weight and be healthy, it's up to you! You're going to have to love this weight off of me." He hears our cries, and he will show us the way and rescue us!

This reminds me of when God was about to free the Israelites from slavery in Egypt. They were stuck and many of them had never known anything else but being a slave. But they cried out to God and He heard them, and He provided their deliverance! Let's read Exodus 6:5-8:

"Now, I have heard their painful cries. I know that they are slaves in Egypt. And I remember my agreement. 6 So tell the Israelites that I say to them, 'I am the Lord. I will save you... I will use my great power to make you free... 7 ...I am the Lord your God, and you will know that I made you free from Egypt. 8 I made a great promise to Abraham, Isaac, and Jacob. I promised to give them a special land. So I will lead you to that land. I will give you that land. It will be yours. I am the Lord'" (ERV).

Notice how many times "I am" and "I will" is mentioned here. God says, "I am the Lord. I will save you. I will make you free. I will lead you! I will give you that land!" Do we deliver ourselves? No. He does it! Scripture says that He is the same yesterday, today and forever (Hebrews 13:8). If He heard the cries for freedom from the Israelites and led them in their Exodus out of slavery and to the Promised Land, He has heard your cries and will also lead you out and into the promised land of a healthy life!

Prayer: Jesus, I thank You that there is a path for me that will work, and You are revealing it to my heart and my mind. I know You love me, and it's Your will that I am healthy. Thank you, Jesus, that You are leading me out and into the promised land of health and vitality.

Say this with me, "Jesus, if I am ever going to lose weight and maintain it, You're going to have to love the weight off of me." Take time today to talk to Jesus about one decision, one change that would help you toward your goal of being healthy. Capture what He ministers to your heart:

Week 5

Gwen Myrie

Day 13

You're Not Defined by Your Failures

"There is therefore now no condemnation to those who are in Christ Jesus..."

– Romans 8:1 NKJV

I remember clearly the day that the words from this scripture penetrated my heart. I was riding in the car with my good friend, Connie, and the Holy Spirit spoke to my heart while we were talking. He sweetly reminded me by saying, "Gwen, there is therefore now no condemnation to those who are in Christ Jesus." I knew immediately what He was referring to. You see, in my heart, I believed that I was a failure. My identity was a failure with a big fat F!

The reason I believed I was a failure was because I would start a weight loss program and see a measure of success, but in the back of my mind (and all along the way) I would hear those accusing voices that would say to me, "You know you're not going to stick with this. The last time you tried losing weight, you didn't last a good month before you gave up! You never finish anything you start, why should anyone believe you this time? You don't even believe in yourself!"

Those accusing voices would taunt me like bullies on a playground assaulting a defenseless kid. "You are a failure, don't embarrass yourself by even trying. You are a loser!" They had defined me for so many years of my life.

The instant the Lord spoke this word to my heart, "Gwen there is no condemnation for all the times you have failed,"

I saw the truth clearly. Up until that time, it had never occurred to me that I was caught in the cycle of defeat by defining myself as a failure. I was living under the condemnation of that lying, accusing voice.

That day, when Jesus spoke to my heart, I thought to myself, *So what if I failed? I don't have to be afraid of failure. I am not defined by how many times I have failed!* The prevailing weight of Jesus' words was my deliverance.

I would attempt losing weight again, knowing in my heart that this time I would succeed! What joy and peace flooded my heart! What strength and courage filled my soul!

In the Passion Translation, Romans 8:1 reads, *"So now the case is closed. There remains no accusing voice of condemnation against those who are joined in life-union with Jesus, the Anointed One."*

Those who are joined in life-union with Jesus are freed from the accusing voice of condemnation. We all know what that voice sounds like. It leaves you feeling powerless to do anything about the problems you are facing, namely, the mountain of weight!

It can be overwhelming and frustrating, but Jesus has done something so powerful and life-altering that enables us to walk boldly into glorious liberty!

Let's look at two explosive verses in Colossians 2:14-15:

"He canceled out every legal violation we had on our record and the old arrest warrant that stood to indict us. He erased it all—our sins, our stained soul—he deleted it all and they cannot be retrieved! Everything we once were in Adam

has been placed onto his cross and nailed permanently there as a public display of cancellation.

"15 Then Jesus made a public spectacle of all the powers and principalities of darkness, stripping away from them every weapon and all their spiritual authority and power to accuse us. And by the power of the cross, Jesus led them around as prisoners in a procession of triumph. He was not their prisoner; they were his!" (TPT).

Every accusing voice that has ever spoken against you to condemn you has been silenced by the power of His cross. Jesus stripped away every weapon from all the powers and principalities of darkness, as well as all their spiritual authority and power to ever accuse you and me again!

He erased it all—our sins, our stained soul—he deleted it all and they cannot be retrieved! Oh, what glorious good news! All those accusing voices that mocked me for so many years of my life have been terminated!

Now I understand Isaiah 54:17: *"'No weapon formed against you shall prosper, And every tongue which rises against you in judgment You shall condemn. This is the heritage of the servants of the Lord, And their righteousness is from Me,' Says the Lord"* (NKJV).

Every condemning and accusing tongue against you and me, our Jesus has silenced permanently! We live in life-union with the risen Savior and the only voice we want to hear is His!

Hear him speak these words to your heart, "There is therefore now no condemnation for all your failures, My beloved one. Will you let My love define you?"

Prayer: Father, thank You for silencing all the accusing voices that have plagued me my entire life and have kept me in a cycle of defeat. By the blood of Your cross, I have been set free from sin and a stained soul. Thank You for showing me that I am defined by Your great love and not by my failures! Now I am ready to let go and let You love the weight off of me.

How does your heart feel knowing that every accusing voice that condemned you has been terminated? Can you identify the lies you have believed concerning your situation? Take a moment, while in the presence of love, and talk to Jesus about those lies. He is here to empower you to live by His definition of who you are. You are defined by His every word!

_____

_____

_____

_____

_____

_____

_____

_____

_____

_____

_____

_____

_____

_____

_____

_____

_____

_____

_____

_____

_____

_____

_____

_____

Day 14

Understand Your Value—You are Worthy

"Knowing that you were not redeemed with corruptible things, like silver or gold, from your aimless conduct received by tradition from your fathers, 19 but with the precious blood of Christ, as of a lamb without blemish and without spot."

— 1 Peter 1:18-19 NKJV

For so many years, I lived with a sense that I was not valuable; that I wasn't worth the time or trouble of anyone. Growing up, I felt like I was everyone's personal dump site. I didn't know there was any other way to live. As a young person, I was told that I wasn't going to amount to anything, and I was good for nothing.

Those words left me feeling as though they were true, because those words shaped my life. I couldn't seem to rise above the words that had been spoken over me by the ones who I thought knew me best. I believed those words, so my life began to unfold as a self-fulfilling prophesy. I didn't discover my value and worth until I became a Christian later in my life.

1 Peter 1:18-19 tells us we were not redeemed with silver or gold but with the precious blood of Christ. The priceless blood of Christ! Silver and gold represent perishable things—things that rust or tarnish in this life, that have no weight or value. My life was so valuable to Jesus, that He

gave the only thing of priceless value—His blood. He held nothing back to prove to me my value and worth!

Blood represents life and His life is the value of my life to Him! By Jesus being willing to die for you, it speaks volumes of your value and worth to Him. You are not a nobody. You are a masterpiece, and Jesus was willing to give up His life in order to purchase you. Let that sink in!

You are the pearl of great price that He gave all that He owned to buy the field where circumstances and troubles buried you. At this point, I am sure you can see your value and worth. But you may be thinking, "How is this connected with letting Jesus love the weight off of me?"

You see, when you don't see yourself as valuable, you will not value what Jesus gave His life to save. He didn't just die for your spiritual life, He died for your physical life as well. When you truly see the price Jesus paid in order for your body to be healthy and strong, you'll begin to show reverence for the body He gave his life to save. He is the Savior of your body as well.

Ephesians 5:23 says, *"For a husband is the head of his wife as Christ is the head of the church. He is the Savior of his body, the church"* (NLT).

Loving who Jesus made you will be one of your greatest delights! Psalms 139:13-14 tells of the delight of our good Father when He was making you.

Let's read it: *"For You formed my innermost parts; You knit me [together] in my mother's womb. I will give thanks and praise to You, for I am fearfully and wonderfully made; Wonderful are Your works, And my soul knows it very well"* (AMP).

Jesus lovingly formed your innermost parts. He knit you together in your mother's womb! He is the one who says that you are fearfully and wonderfully made. Right now, Jesus is asking you to believe what He says about you. Not when you lose the weight, but right now, in this moment, He wants you to believe that you are wonderful.

I was amazed when I looked up the meaning of the word "fearfully" and it means "to stand in awe of; be awed; to cause astonishment and awe; be held in awe." [vi] Can you imagine, this is Jesus' reaction when He made you? He is in awe of you—you are astonishing to Him! This thrills my heart!

Let's look at the word "awe." Some synonyms of this word are "wonder, wonderment, amazement, astonishment, admiration, reverence, and respect." [vii] All of these words describe how you affect the heart of Jesus, your Creator. He thinks and believes the very best and highest thoughts about you and your body! So, the One who made you stands in awe of you! This is such wonderful news to the believing heart. Receive this amazing truth and let it penetrate to the core of your being.

Now let's look at the word "wonderfully." It means "to be distinct, be separated, be distinguished, to be wonderful." [viii] Jesus wanted you! Yes, you! He distinguished you from all other created beings. You are one of a kind! There will never be another you—ever! Everything about you is unique and special, including your body.

Right now, Jesus is loving the weight off of you by telling you the truth. This is what He believes about your body. You are worth far more than rubies or diamonds. Your worth far outweighs any amount of gold. When your heart sees and believes the beauty Jesus sees in you, you'll see your value and worth through His eyes. His love for you will cause you to rest as you let Jesus love the weight off of you!

Prayer: Jesus, I thank You for helping me to see what You saw when You formed me in my mother's womb. Thank You for helping me to believe that I am fearfully and wonderfully made, no matter how much I weigh because my weight doesn't determine my value. Help me to embrace what You say about me. Persuade my heart of Your love for me by revealing to me my value and worth through Your eyes.

How does it make your heart feel knowing that Jesus sees you as valuable and worthy? What are some of the lies that you have believed in this area? Write them down and talk with Jesus about how these lies make your heart feel. How does knowing that you are beautiful to Jesus change the way you see yourself? You are fearfully and wonderfully made!

Day 15

Whose House Is This Anyway?

"You should know that your body is a temple for the Holy Spirit who is in you. You have received the Holy Spirit from God. So you do not belong to yourselves, ²⁰ because you were bought by God for a price. So honor God with your bodies."

– 1 Corinthians 6:19-20 NCV

This scripture was brought to my attention during a time when I was suffering in my body. I remember standing at the kitchen sink when the Holy Spirit whispered this verse to me saying, "Your body is the temple of the Holy Spirit, you are not your own, you have been bought with a price."

At first, I didn't catch on, but Perfect Love repeated it. I heard Him and immediately, I started thinking like a slave. *So, I am not my own, I have a master now?* I used to cringe at the thought of this verse because it conjured up images of slavery. As a black person, I didn't want to be owned by anyone—not even the Lord!

You can imagine my shock and surprise when the Lord ignored my train of thought and sweetly corrected me by showing me His perspective. He said to me, "Do you know what this verse means? 'You are not your own.'" In a loving voice, He went on to say, "I paid the price to be the legal owner of this house."

I was reminded of the verse in 1 Peter 1:18-19: *"God paid a ransom to save you from the impossible road to heaven which*

93

your fathers tried to take, and the ransom he paid was not mere gold or silver as you very well know. ¹⁹ *But he paid for you with the precious lifeblood of Christ, the sinless, spotless Lamb of God"* (TLB).

Then He spoke the most transforming and life-changing words to my heart. "Since I paid for this home, I am responsible for the upkeep and I will make all the necessary repairs." Like lightening, I comprehended what He was saying to me, and in that instant, years of wrong thinking was erased.

I no longer viewed myself as someone else's slave or as a piece of dilapidated property! He set me free to know that He was the owner, therefore, He was responsible for the upkeep of His home. I begin to rejoice in this profound truth, and from that day until now, my body is healing and coming into alignment with that word He spoke to me. I have applied this truth to the area of losing weight as well. The Holy Spirit has led me to eat certain foods that will nourish and strengthen His body!

The Holy Spirit is here to help us and will teach us to honor God with our bodies. Honoring God is showing respect for the wonderful creation that He has made. Our bodies are vital to our existence in this physical world. God desires to live with us and share His life of love, joy, peace and goodness with us every day. He purchased our bodies in order to live with us! Everything Love does is for the object of its affections—you! He can only be good to you. Oh, how He loves to be with you and me! Oh, how He loves us!

2 Corinthians 6:16 says, *"What friendship does God's temple have with demons* [idols]*? For indeed, we are the temple of the living God, just as God has said: I will make*

my home in them and walk among them. I will be their God, and they will be my people" (TPT, brackets added).

God's purpose for making your body was to make you His resting place and sanctuary. God wanted to come home. You are His perfect home, and He is pleased to live in you because He has made you one with Him. Did you know that you are God's address?

When I began to believe that I am God's home, I desired to honor Him by asking Him to work in me. Philippians 2:13 says, *"God is the one who enables you both to want and to actually live out his good purposes"* (CEB).

God is the one who enables us to both want to and to actually live out his good purposes for our lives. He is the one who puts the desire in our hearts to honor Him with our bodies. He will empower you to believe what He believes about your body, and you'll begin to see the desires of your heart effortlessly manifest in your physical body!

I hear the Lord saying, *"For I know the thoughts and plans that I have for you, says the Lord, thoughts and plans for welfare and peace and not for evil, to give you hope in your final outcome"'* (Jeremiah 29:11 AMPC).

Prayer: Father, I thank You for showing me Your design and purpose for my body. You desired to come home. I was created for this purpose. I am Your perfect resting place, Your home. You are responsible for Your home, and You will make all the necessary repairs in me. Thank You for working in me by empowering me to desire what You desire for Your home and for causing me to live out Your good purposes for this body. I believe that Your thoughts and plans for me are good, and they will succeed and prosper in me!

Take time to consider the amazing and incredible creation God has made you. Allow Him to reveal His great passionate love for you through making you His home. How does it make you feel to know that He is responsible for His home, and He will make all the necessary repairs? Today, invite Him to create in you the desire and power to carry out His purpose in you.

_____
_____
_____
_____
_____
_____
_____
_____
_____
_____
_____
_____
_____
_____
_____
_____
_____
_____
_____
_____
_____
_____
_____
_____

Week 6

Connie Witter

Day 16: There's Nothing at All Wrong with You

Day 17: We Will Do It Together

Day 18: Healthy by Design

Day 16

There's Nothing at All Wrong with You

"My darling, everything about you is beautiful, and there is nothing at all wrong with you."

– Jesus, Song of Songs 4:7 NCV

The Song of Songs is one of the most beautiful books in the Bible. It truly is the greatest love story ever told. It reveals Jesus' love song to you.

Zephaniah 3:17 says, *"The Lord your God is in the midst of you, a Mighty One, a Savior [Who saves]! He will rejoice over you with joy; He will rest [in silent satisfaction] and in His love He will be silent and make no mention [of past sins, or even recall them]; He will exult over you with singing"* (AMPC).

This Scripture is one of my favorite verses. The thought of Jesus rejoicing over me with songs of love, and never mentioning my faults or failures, has always brought such peace to my heart. But when I understood that the song He sang over us was actually written out in the Song of Songs, I could finally listen to His song of love by reading it right out of my Bible. Anytime I begin thinking negatively about myself or I just need to be loved, I remember what Jesus sings over me in the Song of Songs. Often, I will go right to Song of Songs 4:7, and let Jesus love me through this verse.

Take a moment to listen to Jesus sing His love song over you again: "My darling, everything about you is beautiful, and there is nothing at all wrong with you!"

For many years of my life, the devil deceived me into believing the lie that there was something wrong with me. This lie kept me disappointed with myself for many years. It was so deeply embedded within my heart that even though I was not aware of it, it was negatively affecting every area of my life. The lie—there's something wrong with you—is often disguised in our analytical questions about ourselves:

Why can't I lose weight?

Why do I continue to fail?

Why do I feel so sad and discouraged?

Why do I struggle in this area of my life?

Every time we look at our failures, or the areas of our lives where we feel like we don't measure up, the voice of condemnation speaks this lie to our hearts: "There's something wrong with you!"

The very root of condemnation is the belief that there's something wrong with you. One day, while I was sharing this with my good friend, Gwen, she said to me, "Connie, since you've been teaching on Song of Songs 4:7, I have realized this is the lie that I have always believed about myself: 'Why can't I lose weight? What is wrong with me?' This lie has held me in bondage for far too long." Shortly after that conversation, Gwen began her journey of letting Jesus love the weight off of her by embracing her true identity in this area of her life.

We have all at one time or another been deceived by this lie that something is wrong with us! It's so subtle that you might not even recognize it. But if there is an area of your life in which you've been disappointed with yourself, I can guarantee this lie is lurking deep within your heart.

Your good Father had a plan from the beginning of time to rescue you from this accusing voice of condemnation. He never wanted you to define yourself by any other voice but His. He wants you to find your identity in His Perfect Love—His never-changing good opinion of you in Christ.

Jesus cleanses your heart from all condemnation with His words of love to you. His word is living water upon your heart, washing away all the lies you've believed about yourself.

Ephesians 5:26-27 says, *"...Christ used the word to make the church clean by washing it with water. ²⁷ He died so that he could give the church to himself like a bride in all her beauty. He died so that the church could be pure and without fault, with no evil or sin or any other wrong thing in it"* (NCV).

It's time for freedom! It's time to let Jesus love the weight of condemnation off of you! It's time that the very root of condemnation that has kept you in bondage to this struggle with your weight be uprooted and completely eliminated from your heart.

It reminds me of the movie *Terminator*. The Terminator came back to destroy what was killing mankind. That's what Jesus did! Condemnation was killing mankind, and Jesus came and terminated condemnation by nailing every accusing voice against you to the cross (Colossians 2:14-15).

Romans 8:1 says, *"So now the case is closed. There remains no accusing voice of condemnation against those who are joined in life-union with Jesus"* (TPT).

Jesus nailed that lying, accusing voice of condemnation that says, "There's something wrong with you," to the cross. Now you are free to let Jesus love the weight off of you by embracing His voice of Truth and agreeing with what He says about you!

So, don't let that lie hold you in bondage for one more day! The next time you hear that accusing voice of condemnation trying to get you to believe, "What's wrong with me?" Boldly respond the same way Jesus did: "It is written, Truth has spoken, and there is nothing at all wrong with Me! Condemnation you have been terminated!"

Prayer: Jesus, I'm ready to let You love this weight off of me! Thank You for cleansing my heart from every lie I've believed about myself that has held me in bondage to this struggle to lose weight. What You say about me is true! Everything about me is beautiful, and there's nothing at all wrong with me! Your love has set me free!

How does it make your heart feel to hear Jesus say, "My darling, everything about you is beautiful and there is nothing at all wrong with you?" Take time today to respond to His words of love to you. Let His Love define who you are.

_____

_____

_____

_____

_____

_____

_____

_____

_____

_____

_____

_____

_____

_____

_____

_____

_____

_____

_____

_____

_____

_____

_____

_____

_____

_____

_____

_____

_____

Day 17

We Will Do It Together

"You must catch the troubling foxes, those sly little foxes that hinder our relationship... Will you catch them and remove them for Me? We will do it together."

— Song of Songs 2:15 TPT

In Song of Songs 2:8-15, we read about how we, as the bride of Christ, hear our bridegroom's voice coming to us, speaking and singing songs of love and freedom. He leaps with joy over the mountains and hills to the places of your heart where you have taken on a different opinion of yourself then His. He peers through the portal of your soul, and He sees those areas where you are hiding behind the lies you have believed about yourself, and yet He continues to pursue you and sing His love song over you—beckoning you to come out of your hiding place.

Listen to how Jesus, your bridegroom, speaks to you as He peers through the portal of your soul and sees the areas where you are hiding behind shame. Listen to His words of love, reminding you how He sees you, awakening your heart to His glorious plan to live as one with you:

"The one I love calls to me: Arise, my dearest. Hurry, my darling. Come away with me! I have come as you have asked to draw you to my heart and lead you out. For now is the time, my beautiful one. [11] The season has changed, the bondage of your barren winter has ended, and the season of hiding is over and gone...

"13 ...The budding vines of new life are now blooming everywhere. The fragrance of their flowers whispers, 'There is change in the air.' Arise, my love, my beautiful companion, and run with me to the higher place. For now is the time to arise and come away with Me.

"15 You must catch the troubling foxes, those sly little foxes that hinder our relationship. For they raid our budding vineyard of love to ruin what I've planted within you. Will you catch them and remove them for Me? We will do it together" (Song of Songs 2:10-11, 13, & 15 TPT).

Jesus comes to the places of your heart where you are hiding behind guilt and shame. These are the troubling foxes that we hold onto at times that hinder Jesus from living fully through us. Jesus, your bridegroom, has come as you have asked to draw you to His heart and lead you out of the dark places of your soul.

He says, "Now is the time for you to experience the freedom I paid such a great price for you to walk in. Shame has held you in bondage and kept you in the season of 'your barren winter,' a place where the fruit of righteousness has not manifested. But today is the day of salvation, now is the time for that fruit to come forth. There is change in the air. Let my love transform that area of your life that has been barren—where the seed I've planted in you has not yet blossomed. It's time, My love, for you to come to the higher place with me. It is time for My glory to shine through you in this area of your life."

Jesus says that in order for His glory to shine through you, you must catch those troubling foxes that hinder your relationship with Him. They raid your vineyard of love and ruin what He has planted within you. You can recognize the foxes by the negative emotions that come up in your heart. He says, "Come to Me in those moments and we will get rid of the foxes together."

Despite your feelings of failure and hopelessness, Jesus continues to tell you how He sees you.

In Song of Songs 4:1 & 4, Jesus says, *"Listen, my dearest darling, you are so beautiful—you are beauty itself to me!... 4 When I look at you, I see your inner strength, so stately and strong. You are as secure as David's fortress. Your virtues and grace cause a thousand famous soldiers to surrender to your beauty"* (TPT).

In these verses, Jesus is opening your eyes to the truth of your true identity in Him. Jesus sees you as one with Him. He speaks to you and reminds you who you truly are as His bride! He sees you as He sees Himself! One with Him—His equal—His bride! In my personal journey to freedom, when I began to say, "Yes," to Jesus and the words of love He spoke over me, those foxes of doubt and shame that were in my heart died, and my life began to reflect His glory.

In Song of Songs 4:6, you can see that when you come into agreement with Jesus and what He sings over you, that's when true transformation and freedom begin to happen in your life.

The bride says, *"I've made up my mind. Until the darkness disappears and the dawn has fully come, in spite of shadows and fears, I will go to the mountain top with you—the mountain of suffering love and the hill of burning incense. Yes, I will be Your bride"* (TPT).

The moment you make up your mind to live as the bride of the King and say, "YES!" to how He sees you, you begin to reign victorious in life. It is then that you experience what Jesus promised you: "We will get rid of the foxes together!" Jesus has already said "Yes!" to you. When you say, "Yes!" to Him, His glory will manifest in your life!

2 Corinthians 1:20 says, *"The yes to all of God's promises is in Christ, and through Christ we say yes to the glory of God"* (NCV).

Prayer: I will go to the mountain top with You, Jesus! I say, "Yes" to everything You say about me! I'm ready for the foxes to be gone so that my life will bear the fruit of Your glory. We will do it together! I trust You because I know You love me! Yes, I will be Your bride. I will live as one with You!

Take a moment to talk to Jesus about the troubling foxes that have hindered you from experiencing the fruit of God's glory in your life. How does it make you feel to hear Jesus say, "We will get rid of the foxes together?" He has already said, "Yes!" to you! Take some time today to say, "Yes!" to what He says about you and watch as His glory manifests in your life.

_____

_____

_____

_____

_____

_____

_____

_____

_____

_____

_____

_____

_____

_____

_____

_____

_____

_____

_____

_____

_____

_____

_____

_____

Day 18

Healthy by Design

"Beloved, I wish above all things that thou mayest prosper and be in health, even as thy soul prospereth."

— 3 John 2 KJV

I have always loved this verse. It reveals the heart of our good Father and His will for all of His children. You are His beloved child, and He wishes above all things that you would prosper in every way, and that includes a healthy body and a healthy mind.

I have a friend who recently shared how his eating habits had taken a toll on his health. Even though he knew it was the Father's will for him to be strong and healthy, and even though he had ministered healing to many people through his ministry, years of overeating and unhealthy eating habits had brought an extra 40-50 pounds on his frame and had wreaked havoc on his body. He had been diagnosed with type 2 diabetes and high blood pressure, and it was destroying his health. He shared how he knew this was not His Father's will for him, and it was time that he began to walk in the fullness of life that Jesus came to give him.

I watched as Jesus began to help him make healthy choices. He transformed before my eyes as the extra 45 pounds melted off of his body. Within months, his type 2 diabetes was gone, and his blood pressure was normal. He began walking daily, increasing his distance until he was walking several miles a day. Wow! I saw life come back into him, and it was so beautiful to see! What our good Father wishes for all of His children began to manifest in his body. As he began to see himself as a strong and healthy man, healthy choices became his lifestyle.

You were designed by God to be healthy and strong in your body and in your mind. It is never His will for any of His children to be at an unhealthy weight. If overeating and unhealthy eating habits have caused you to experience sickness or pain in your body, you don't have to stay there. Jesus is in you, and He has promised to help you and restore your health. Take a moment to remember the benefits of being a beloved child of God!

Psalm 103:2-5 says, *"Bless the Lord, O my soul; And forget not all His benefits: 3 Who forgives all your iniquities, Who heals all your diseases, 4 Who redeems your life from destruction, Who crowns you with loving-kindness and tender mercies, 5 Who satisfies your mouth with good things, So that your youth is renewed like the eagle's"* (NKJV).

Did you hear that? Jesus forgives all your past unhealthy choices! They are forgiven and forgotten! He heals all the symptoms in your body that were caused by those unhealthy choices. Today is the day of salvation! His mercy is new every morning! It's never too late to begin to trust Him to help you make healthy choices so that you can enjoy your life to the fullest. It's never too late to begin to see yourself the way He sees you!

When you're ready to say, "Yes" to what He says about you, He is there to redeem your life from destruction, for He crowns you with His unfailing love and compassion. He is not disappointed with you. You are the delight of His heart. He only wants to rescue you from the troubling foxes of guilt and shame that have kept you believing the lie that you deserve to be unhealthy because of the choices you have made. That's not true! Whatever havoc has been done to your body, Jesus is ready to redeem and restore. He is your wonderful Savior, and He loves you!

Psalm 103:5 reminds me of my friend and his journey to health. It says Jesus satisfies your mouth with good things so that your youth is renewed like the eagle's. Not only did Jesus satisfy my friend's mouth with good, healthy food that brought nourishment and health to his body, but after he lost those 45 extra pounds, he literally looked 10 years younger! His youth was renewed like the eagle's, just like this verse promised!

Your body was magnificently created by your good Father to heal and restore. You were designed for health and wholeness. That's who you really are! When you believe this truth, that's when restoration and healing begin. The amazing thing about my friend is that it took years for unhealthy choices to wreak havoc on his body, but it only took a few short months of believing the truth about himself to begin to experience more energy, health and vitality. Jesus will restore the years that the canker worm has stolen and cause your body to vibrate with health as you embrace the benefits of being His beloved child.

When your good Father looks at you, He sees you healthy and whole in Jesus. Today is the day to begin to see yourself that way too! You are one with Perfect Health! It's time to leave your past behind and begin to live the healthy life Jesus created you to live! You are worth it!

Prayer: Father, You designed me to be healthy and whole. I am ready to let You do the work in my heart necessary for me to experience a healthy weight for my body. Today is a new day, and I receive Your love and grace to restore the years that have been stolen from me and bring forth health and vitality in my body! You forgive all my sins and heal all my diseases! You redeem my life from destruction and crown me with loving-kindness. You satisfy My mouth with good things so that my youth is renewed like the eagle's! Thank You for restoring my life with Your love!

Take a moment to reflect on what your good Father spoke to your heart today. Make Psalm 103:2-5 personal. How do the benefits of being His child bring hope to your heart?

_____

_____

_____

_____

_____

_____

_____

_____

_____

_____

_____

_____

_____

_____

_____

_____

_____

_____

_____

_____

_____

_____

_____

_____

_____

_____

Week 7

Sherry Riether

Day 19: **Overwhelmed No More**

Day 20: **You Lack Nothing**

Day 21: **From Bondage to Freedom**

Day 19

Overwhelmed No More

"Give your entire attention to what God is doing right now, and don't get worked up about what may or may not happen tomorrow. God will help you deal with whatever hard things come up when the time comes."

– Matthew 6:34 MSG

When you think about the amount of weight you need to lose, does it overwhelm you? Does it bring thoughts of defeat? It did to me. I needed to lose almost 90 pounds. Ninety! When I would think about that amount, it wasn't long before condemning and defeating thoughts would start to creep into my mind. *How did I ever get to this point? It's hopeless, you're so far gone that there is no way back now. You're just going to have to live being fat.* Even if I got my resolve back, that I was going to lose the weight no matter what, panic would set in—90 pounds? *How can I lose 90 pounds?!*

Thoughts like that used to have me defeated and overwhelmed. But God is so good! As I daily declared the truth over myself, often the Holy Spirit would drop another word in my heart that would become a building block of success for me.

One day, when I was talking to Jesus about my weight, I heard Him say these words to me, "You don't have to lose weight next year, next month, next week or even tomorrow.

All you have to do is focus on this one decision right now to be healthy."

What? Just focus on one decision right now? "Focus on making one choice, one decision," Jesus said to me. "You can do it! Just focus on one."

It reminded me of Philippians 4:13: *"I can do all things through Christ who strengthens me"* (NKJV).

I began thinking about what making one choice, one decision meant. It meant that, through Jesus, I can do all things! Losing weight and getting healthy really is about making one healthy decision at a time. That's all. Maybe this is nothing new to you, but for me it was a revelation! As I meditated on the one decision, Jesus helped me to see that I could do it!

This helped me so many times as I began to change my eating habits and started exercising. When I would have a difficult day, I would declare, "I don't have to lose weight next year, next month, next week, or even tomorrow. All I have to do is focus on making a healthy decision today."

Focus on one day? I can do anything for a day! Jesus was loving the weight off of me by changing my thoughts toward goal-setting and some of those goals got down to making a healthy choice moment-by-moment!

There were times when I even said to myself, "I don't have to lose weight today, this evening or this afternoon! All I have to do is make this one healthy choice in this moment, right now." Breaking it down like that suddenly made weight loss less overwhelming.

Don't worry about tomorrow! Focus on what God is doing right now to help you!

"But Sherry, not worrying about losing weight is how I ended up overweight in the first place! How can I not worry about it?"

Worrying is to be anxious with cares. We can get so caught up in everything we have to do that we get nothing done! Worrying gets us into thought patterns that lead us into fear and feelings of being overwhelmed which can cripple us. Jesus tells us to give our entire attention to God —what He's doing right now. Why? Because God is good! He only has good for us and toward us.

Before Jesus tells you not to worry about tomorrow, He tells you the Father knows what you need and to seek first the kingdom of God and His righteousness (Matt 6:33-34). Your good Father knows what you need to help you make changes in your life. He helps you by His Grace!

Grace is the divine influence upon your heart and its reflection in your life. Losing weight can be overwhelming, but He has a plan that will work for you. As you turn your heart to Him, He influences you toward ways that are healthy.

Weight loss goals can seem like a mountain. Whether you need to lose 90 pounds, or that last 9 pounds, or the 19 pounds you regained. Let him gently and lovingly influence your heart and you will see the path forward! It's a path of victory because God is good! He already knows what you need to be successful! That's why you don't have to worry about tomorrow! That mountain will come down!

Let Jesus Love the Weight off of You

Zechariah 4:7 says, *"Who are you, O great mountain? Before Zerubbabel, you shall become a plain! And he shall bring forth the capstone with shouts of 'Grace, grace to it!'"* (NKJV).

Focus on what God is doing in your heart right now. Shout grace to that mountain, and He will lead you in triumph!

Prayer: Jesus, thank You that I do not have to lose weight next year, next month, or even tomorrow. Thank You for helping me focus on what You are doing in my heart right now. I shout grace to this mountain, and it will overwhelm me no more! Amen!

When you focus on Jesus helping you make "one choice, one decision," how does that influence you to not worry about tomorrow? Take time today to let God minister to your heart and let Jesus love the weight off of you!

_____

_____

_____

_____

_____

_____

_____

_____

_____

_____

_____

_____

_____

_____

_____

_____

_____

_____

_____

_____

_____

_____

_____

_____

_____

_____

_____

_____

_____

_____

Day 20

You Lack Nothing

"The Lord is my Shepherd, I lack nothing."

– Psalm 23:1 NIV

I read an article in a popular psychology magazine. It's not my normal pastime, but I have always been curious about why people act, think, and behave the way that they do. Mostly because I want to understand why I act, think, and behave the way that I do. For example, why was I an emotional eater? Some people say they eat when they are depressed, or happy, or nervous—I can eat no matter what emotion I am experiencing!

Anyway, this article was fascinating to me because the author, probably without knowing it, was confirming what Proverbs 23:7 says: *"As he thinks in his heart, so is he"* (NKJV). In other words, we experience what we believe.

The author said that the way we perceive our reality is determined by our beliefs. He also said that basic core beliefs that spring from behaviors and attitudes we experienced as children are often accepted as facts. These "facts" become the truths out of which we live.

Psychologists would say these truths are like programs that become hard-wired within our subconscious. It's out of these truths that our beliefs are generated, and our beliefs drive our behaviors and attitudes. As adults, these programs are still running in our lives even though they may make no sense, may limit our expectations, and may even be detrimental to our well-being.

As I thought about the article, I realized some "facts" I had believed as a child were incorrect "truths" that had influenced me all my life. I grew up in a home where we constantly struggled to pay the bills. Every financial decision was met with, "We can't afford it." I learned early on not to ask my parents for money because of the stress it brought them.

Don't get me wrong, they never blamed me for the financial position we were in, but I took on that identity of lack. It was not until later in life that I realized just how much of a grip this sense of lack had on me and how much it impacted the way I lived.

Food, on the other hand, was not lacking. Family meals were a big part of our lives and became a source of comfort. But even though there was abundance in quantity, we learned to abide by the common household saying of "clean your plate" because we didn't want to waste anything. In a way, even that seemed to reinforce a sense of lack in me through my childhood years. Turning to food for comfort was almost a given. I became just like many in my family— an emotional eater and overweight.

The Bible makes it clear that our thinking and our hearts are inseparably linked. This is what Proverbs 4:23 tells us. *"Be careful how you think; your life is shaped by your thoughts"* (GNT).

What we think affects our heart. Likewise, the condition of our heart affects our thinking. We experience what we think. We experience what we believe. If we think we lack, then we will act out of that heart condition and various symptoms will present themselves in our lives. If you have a heart belief of lack, you can end up being stingy with your finances or enter into overeating to compensate for the lack you are feeling. I did both.

A few years ago, I realized lack had become my identity. I was listening to a message when the Father spoke to my heart and said, "You need to let Me Father you."

I said, "What do you mean, God? I do believe that You are my Father."

God spoke to my heart again and said, "You think of Me as a Father, but you do not believe I will Father you."

Still confused, I asked God to explain what He meant. I will never forget what He said.

"You think of Me as a Father, but you do not trust I will take care of you. You really don't believe that I am your Shepherd who won't let you suffer any lack. You don't trust me to Father you."

In that moment, I broke down in tears. It was true. I had not let my guard down to be fully vulnerable to God as my Father. I didn't trust that I could completely rely on Him for everything. I had relied on myself to take care of me. I believed in lack and that lack had held such a grip on my life that I turned to food as a comforter instead of turning to my Father.

I thought about what He had shown me and said, "You're right, God. I have not let You Father me. I want to, but I don't know how. You're going to have to help me surrender to Your Fathering." Peace immediately began to settle into my heart and the crippling grip of lack was broken. It changed how I gave in my finances and it changed how I looked at food.

When I would pay a bill, I would say, "Thank You, Father. There is plenty more where that came from because You are my Shepherd and I suffer no lack." Then I applied it to eating. Instead of piling my plate with large portions, I began to choose smaller portions and would say, "There is plenty to eat. I can eat this, and if I am really hungry afterward, I can eat something else." This was such a new and empowering way to live life! I began leaving the mindset of not having enough. I began living out of a belief of having an abundance!

Prayer: Thank You, Father, that You care for us in abundance. You are my shepherd. I suffer no lack! It makes my heart happy and sets my mind to rest that You are a good, good Father, and You Father me so well.

Take time today to meditate on God as your good, good Father. He is your Shepherd and you suffer no lack. How does this empower you to live free from anything in your past that causes you to have a sense of lack?

_____

_____

_____

_____

_____

_____

_____

_____

_____

_____

_____

_____

_____

_____

_____

_____

_____

_____

_____

_____

_____

_____

_____

_____

_____

_____

_____

Day 21

From Bondage to Freedom

"For if by the trespass of the one, death reigned through the one; so much more will those who receive the abundance of grace and of the gift of righteousness reign in life through the one, Jesus Christ."

– Romans 5:17 WEB

Is it possible to reign and rule in the area of weight loss and health? Yes! Can losing weight be as simple as letting Jesus love the weight off of you? Yes!

You may ask, "How can you be so sure?" Because the Word of God says so. God Himself said He is the God that heals (Exodus 15:26) and 2 Corinthians 1:20 tells us that all the promises of God are "Yes", and we get to say "Amen," to them. So, yes, God wants us to be healthy! Therefore, we can believe we can lose weight and we can believe that He provided a way for us to rule and reign in this area!

We all have the desire be healthy—it is in all of us. When we feel that desire rising in our hearts, we can believe that God is already at work in us, not only to bring us out of unhealthy habits, but to set us in a place of victory from which we rule and reign! We are no longer in bondage to old habits and old heart beliefs that cause us to stay slaves to the mentality that poor health and obesity are all there is for us! NO! There is a promised land and He is delivering us to it! Amen!

For most of my adult life I felt like I was trapped in a fat body and there was no way out. It seemed like no matter what I tried, nothing worked, and I tried everything to find a way to freedom. I drank the shakes but was so hungry I only lasted a couple of days before giving up. I took the diet pills, lost a few pounds, but they made me jittery and gave me insomnia. I took the "fat burn" pills and got high blood pressure.

I even reduced my calorie intake to 500 calories a day and gave myself injections of some "natural" hormone that was supposed to help me burn fat while I retained muscle. Wow.... Just writing all of these down makes me realize how desperate I had become about losing weight. No wonder I ended up giving up for a while!

I was so desperate for help, I turned everywhere but to God for hope and answers. I realize now that I was looking to external remedies for an internal problem. I was looking to an external system that would "control" me because I felt out of control.

It wasn't until I began a journey to understand that Christ made me righteous as a gift that I turned to Him for help. That meant that all my sins—past, present and future—were forgiven. There was nothing keeping me from the love of the Father. I received the abundance of grace and I finally was confident that all His promises to me were true. Why had it never occurred to me to trust Jesus for weight loss? I believed for healing, but why not to be at a healthy weight?

One day I just said to Him, "If I am ever going to lose weight it is up to you, Jesus!" I was kind of shocked at the force and sincerity that came out in my voice when I said it. It was definitely a turning point for me. I was done trying to do it on my own, done trying to listen to the world's solutions, done trying to look outside of the One who loves me for the answer! If I wasn't confident and secure in my salvation, I would have likely cowered, expecting God to strike me down for being impertinent.

Not long after I said this, I was at a Women of Grace Conference where Connie Witter was speaking. In the middle of her message, she abruptly stopped and said, "Some of you here today have been struggling with your weight. Let Jesus love the weight off of you!"

Wow! Those words hit my heart like an arrow hitting a bullseye! My heart had been prepared by God for the sound of deliverance. It was time for freedom, and I received it fully! I wasn't sure how it would work out, but I just began agreeing with Jesus' words over me. "I am healthy. I'm at a healthy weight."

I was saying these things before I ever lost one pound, before I ever saw any changes in my body. The Holy Spirit was at work in me when the desire sprung up in my heart. I began to let Jesus love the weight off of me. I was declaring the truth over me based on the promises of God! That's when I began to reign in life!

Letting Jesus love the weight off of you isn't about doing nothing. It's about listening to the One who knows you the best. He knows you better than you know yourself, and He is speaking to your heart right now to show you how to walk in freedom in this area.

You can believe right now that God is already at work! That desire within you is Him working in you and convincing you that you are no longer a slave to being unhealthy. Not only can you believe you can lose the weight, you can believe that you rule and reign through Jesus!

Prayer: Thank You, Jesus, for the gift of Your righteousness. I receive it freely and know that because You put me in right standing with the Father, all of His promises to me are "Yes!" and I say "Amen!" I now rule and reign in the abundance of grace!

All of God's promises are "Yes" in Christ, and we get to say "Amen" to them. Freedom comes when we begin to agree with Jesus. Does knowing this give you hope that you can rule and reign in your health?

_____

_____

_____

_____

_____

_____

_____

_____

_____

_____

_____

_____

_____

_____

_____

_____

_____

_____

_____

_____

_____

_____

_____

_____

_____

_____

_____

_____

_____

_____

_____

Week 8

Gwen Myrie

Day 22: Reigning Through Righteousness

Day 23: So Long Self-Effort

Day 24: Guilt-Free Eating

Day 22

Reigning Through Righteousness

"For if by the one man's offense death reigned through the one, much more those who receive abundance of grace and of the gift of righteousness will reign in life through the One, Jesus Christ."

– Romans 5:17 NKJV

I remember the day I gave up on ever losing weight. I knew that if I were ever to conquer this one area of my life it would take a miracle intervention from God. I'd been so defeated in my attempts to lose the weight that I felt like quitting and just living in an unhealthy, miserable state.

I knew this was no way to live. In fact, I felt as though I was dying on the inside. Back then, I thought God had better things to do than assist me with weight loss. I am so thankful that our Heavenly Father is interested in every area of our lives, and that He cares about everything that concerns us. 1 Peter 5:7 says that we can cast all our cares on Him because He cares for us!

Romans 5:17 is a powerful Scripture to meditate on and ponder because it is the grace of God and the free gift of righteousness that empowers us to reign in this life through our union with Christ Jesus. Grace comes from the Greek word *charis*, and it means "the merciful kindness by which God, exerting his holy influence upon souls, turns them to Christ, keeps, strengthens, increases them in Christian faith, knowledge, affection, and kindles them to the exercise of the Christian virtues."[ix]

Can you see that it is His merciful kindness by which God (not in your own strength or self-effort) exerts His Holy influence upon your soul and turns you to Christ? He does this so that you might be strengthened and increased in faith. He also increases you in the Christian virtues of self-control and goodness. With God all things are possible, even losing weight!

It never crossed my mind that I should be good to myself by respecting this fearfully and wonderfully made creation that our great Creator made me to be! We are such wonderful masterpieces in the eyes of our beautiful Savior. The reason I never associated being good to myself with losing weight was because I believed lies about myself and my body. But when you receive God's grace you are empowered by His Holy Spirit!

When you own the truth that God's desire is to be merciful toward all of your failures, and that He has compassion on you to help you, then you'll rise from the place of hopelessness and despair! You will rise up and be confident in the love of God for you. You will not be afraid anymore of failing or have the desire to give up and quit. The root meaning of grace is "to rejoice, be glad; to rejoice exceedingly; to be well, thrive." [x] This should make you shout for joy! God has an abundance of grace for you!

Now, let us take a look at this powerful word "righteousness". For a long time, I didn't know what this word meant. It was confusing to me until I asked the Lord to reveal what it means to be made righteous. Look at the meaning of this awesome word: "in a broad sense: state of him who is as he ought to be, the condition acceptable to God." [xi]

Did you know that when God looks at you, He sees you as having His very righteousness? Did you know that you are already acceptable to God? You are as you ought to be as far as our Heavenly Father is concerned. That is incredible! God sees you as already perfect in His sight.

You may ask, "How can that be?"

Romans 4:17 says, "(As it is written, 'I have made you a father of many nations') in the presence of Him whom he believed—God, who gives life to the dead and calls those things which do not exist as though they did" (NKJV).

God called Abraham the father of many nations before he had Isaac. God is in the creating business; when He speaks, He is creating. He already knows the truth about you, and when He made you righteous, He said that you are as you ought to be! God says that you are acceptable to Him right now!

Righteousness is a gift that you did not earn. It was provided for you by the death, burial and resurrection of Jesus Christ. Receive His gift of acceptance and approval! Receive the truth that you are as you ought to be in God's eyes and reign through Jesus Christ. Let Jesus love the weight off of you by calling you as He sees you. Reign in life by believing Him!

Prayer: Father, thank You for your abundant provision of grace, Your empowerment by the Holy Spirit to reign in this area of my life. Thank You for the free gift of righteousness! You see me as I ought to be: holy, acceptable, approved and innocent in Your sight because of Jesus. Help me to believe what You see when You look at me. Thank You for loving the weight off of me.

How does it make your heart feel knowing that God cares about you in this area of weight loss? Take time to let God's grace and mercy flood your heart as you think about how perfectly righteous God has made you. Do you see how believing what your good Father says about you will cause you to reign in life?

_____

_____

_____

_____

_____

_____

_____

_____

_____

_____

_____

_____

_____

_____

_____

_____

_____

_____

_____

_____

_____

_____

_____

_____

Day 23

So Long Self-Effort

*"[Not in your own strength] for it is God Who is
all the while effectually at work in you
[energizing and creating in you the power and
desire], both to will and to work for His good
pleasure and satisfaction and delight."*

– Philippians 2:13 AMPC

Not in my own strength! How can that be? There must
be something I have to do. How will the pounds ever fall
off, if I don't do something? That doesn't sound right. That
can't be true. Right? Don't I need an eating plan? Don't I
need to exercise?

Yes! You'll know what to eat and you'll want to get up
and move when you start to shed the weight. But in all
honesty, that is not the problem. The problem is the "doing"
at the expense of "being".

In reality, all diets have the same thing in common: they
employ the same principles. All diets have an eating plan
and an exercise plan. All of them promise the same thing,
and if you want to lose weight, you have to do everything you
are told. There is a proverb that we would do well to heed in
following the path of the world's mindset.

Proverbs 16:25 says, *"Before every person there is a
path that seems like the right one to take, but it leads
straight to hell!"* (TPT).

For a great number of years, I lived in hell trying to follow eating plans and exercising to no avail because the real problem was not physical, but spiritual. I did not believe what my Jesus said about me. I did not know who I was, and that is hell!

At first, all dieting plans sound so good, because with a plan we know what to do. But how many people do you know, after implementing the rules of dieting, were able to maintain it? I have seen some very strong-willed people submit to failure after a few years because they didn't address the reason for the weight gain in the first place.

For those of us who have no will power, we gain all our weight back and then some. Seriously, if you could lose weight by following rules of weight loss coupled with self-effort, you would have been successful by now. These plans seem like the right one, the right way and have the appearance of being effective but they all deal with the outside and not the inside.

Your heart is the place where weight loss begins. If you rely solely on diet plans, you will fail, and deep down you already know this. I can assure you, there is a better way!

Jesus is the better way. He will help you lose the weight without employing the strategies of the dieting world. He knows that failure is programmed into all rule keeping systems, including dieting rules. He knows what it will produce in your heart when you fail. You will feel defeated, hopeless and condemned. Now that's hell!

He knows that the problem is what you're believing and not what you're eating. He knows this is a heart issue. He is the King of hearts, and He knows exactly how to work in you and get to the root of the problem.

Philippians 2:13 is such an amazing verse of scripture, let's read it again: *"[Not in your own strength] for it is God who is all the while effectually at work in you energizing and creating in you the power and desire, both to will and to work for his good pleasure and satisfaction and delight"* (AMPC).

It is God who is all the while effectually at work in you energizing and creating in you the power and desire. Who is at work in you? God (the Father, Son and Holy Spirit) is at work in you. It is not by your might or your power, but it is by His Spirit working in you (Zachariah 4:6).

This reminds me of a beautiful scripture, Song of Songs 2:15. *"You must catch the troubling foxes, those sly little foxes that hinder our relationship. For they raid our budding vineyard of love to ruin what I've planted within you. Will you catch them and remove them for me? We will do it together"* (TPT).

What an amazing reminder that you're not doing this alone. The Lover of your soul is helping you. What happy progress you will make in this journey! Jesus wants you to lean your entire being on Him and trust Him to work in you.

He is energizing you now! He is creating in you the power and the desire to believe that you are successful right now! He is working in you so that you are resolved and determined to be victorious in this area of your life—right now! Jesus is motivating you at this very moment to believe the truth that it is His life that is at work in you.

It is time to get excited about your heart being fully persuaded to believe what Jesus says about you! As your heart is persuaded, you will find that you take delight and joy in the process. He will work in your heart in such a powerful way that will leave you assured of his love! You will truly know what is means to let Jesus love the weight off of you!

Prayer: Father, thank You that it is not in my own strength that I will lose the weight. I believe that You are all the while effectually at work in me. You are energizing and creating in me the power and desire to believe You. Thank You for persuading my heart of Your love for me. Thank You for helping me to get rid of the little foxes that destroy our budding vineyard of love. Thank You for persuading me to believe that You are loving the weight off of me.

Reread Song of Songs 2:15. How does it make your heart feel knowing that Jesus says, "We will do this together?" Take time to sit down and let Jesus love you.

_____

_____

_____

_____

_____

_____

_____

_____

_____

_____

_____

_____

_____

_____

_____

_____

_____

_____

_____

_____

_____

_____

_____

_____

_____

_____

_____

_____

_____

Day 24

Guilt-Free Eating

*"So why would you allow anyone to judge you
because of what you eat or drink..."*

– Colossians 2:16 TPT

When reading this scripture, I thought it was referring to other people judging me. Did you know that you are included with anyone? Don't allow anyone to judge you and don't allow yourself to judge you, either. The word "judge" means to pronounce an opinion concerning right or wrong." [xii]

Don't pronounce an opinion concerning right or wrong over yourself about what you eat or drink. Wow! How many times have we made judgments about foods? How many times have we taken the opinions of the dieting world, the opinions of self-appointed gurus on what is good for you and what is bad (evil)?

God has an opinion as well (we will take a look at His opinion later) but first, when did all judgments about eating and drinking begin?

Genesis 2:16-17 says, *"The Lord God commanded him, "You may eat the fruit from any tree in the garden, ¹⁷ but you must not eat the fruit from the tree which gives the knowledge of good and evil. If you ever eat fruit from that tree, you will die!"* (NCV).

The tree of the knowledge of good and evil is where all eating plans—what is good and what is evil or bad—find their genesis. Someone will ask, "Well, shouldn't we eat good foods?" Who told you what is good? Where did our opinions on what is good and evil come from? The world system is founded on the tree of the knowledge of good and evil. Even some Christian dieting plans employ good and bad foods—they are all from the same polluted source. Everything we think about, with reference to good or bad (evil) has its origin in that tree.

Don't allow anyone to judge you or pronounce an opinion concerning right or wrong in the area of what you eat or drink. The apostle Paul wrote the following exhortation by the Spirit of God to the Colossian church. He wrote God's opinion on eating and drinking, not man's!

In 1 Corinthians 6:12, Paul said, *"'I am allowed to do all things,' but not all things are good for me to do. 'I am allowed to do all things,' but I will not let anything make me its slave'"* (NCV).

When you decide what is good or bad in what you eat, you are bringing yourself under the "Law of Eating and Drinking." When you put yourself under the law of anything, then when you break it, you are subject to the penalty of being under that law.

So, for instance, you think eating cake, ice cream, and sugar (or any junk food) is not good for you. What happens in your heart when you break that law and eat those things? The first thing that happens is what happened to Adam and Eve; they felt fear, shame, and guilt. They felt condemnation.

That's right, when you eat something that is contrary to the "Law of Eating and Drinking," you also feel fear, shame, guilt and condemnation. When you come under the influence of condemnation, you enter the cycle of defeat.

Here are some of the thoughts that will assault your heart: *I can't lose weight, I have no self-control, I am a failure, I am a loser.* These thoughts are judgments that condemn you and put you in the cycle of defeat! You can trace these thoughts back to the tree of the knowledge of good and evil.

God's opinion on eating and drinking should be the only opinion that you consider when eating and drinking. We are led by the Spirit of God in everything, even our food choices. We have self-control because we have God's Spirit who produces this fruit in us.

I can almost hear you asking, "Gwen, are you saying we can eat anything?"

Yes, you can! At the same, time, keep in mind what the apostle Paul said, *"'I am allowed to do all things,' but not all things are good for me to do. 'I am allowed to do all things,' but I will not let anything make me its slave"* (1 Corinthians 6:12 NCV)

Does what you are eating and drinking benefit you? Let this saying in Paul's letter penetrate your heart, "but not all things are good (beneficial) for me to do." Eating four slices of cake doesn't benefit you. Eating a whole bag of chips doesn't benefit you. Drinking a two-liter bottle of Coke doesn't benefit you. Drinking a bottle of wine doesn't benefit you. And thinking, *I am good because I've eaten a healthy salad* doesn't benefit you either!

Remember the tree of the knowledge of good and evil! Whatever you eat or drink should benefit you! Are vegetables delicious to you? Eat them without judging them good or bad! Do you like sweets? Or salty things? Eat them without judging them good or bad! For crying out loud!

EAT WITH NO JUDGEMENT! NO GUILT! EAT IN PEACE!!

Read 1 Timothy 4:4-5: "*...These liars have lied so well and for so long that they've lost their capacity for truth. They will tell you not to get married. They'll tell you not to eat this or that food—perfectly good food God created to be eaten heartily and with thanksgiving by believers who know better! Everything God created is good, and to be received with thanks. Nothing is to be sneered at and thrown out. God's Word and our prayers make every item in creation holy*" (MSG).

Remember, Paul also said, "but I will not let anything make me its slave." How do you stop being a slave to food? Simply make no more judgments about what you are eating and drinking. Jesus will help you to eat this way.

Remember, when you pronounce a judgment of whether something is good or bad, you are implementing the "Law of Eating and Drinking." When you come under any law, failure is inevitable. Defeat, frustration, and hopelessness are the fruit of the law.

Jesus has set you free from the law by nailing it to His cross! Jesus has set us free from all judgment! We are completely free, not partially free! Let no man take you captive by any rule keeping system! Let Jesus show you the way to guilt-free eating as He loves the weight off of you!

Prayer: Jesus, help me to remove all judgments about food. I receive Your opinion about food. Thank You for helping me choose what benefits my body, Your temple. You have delivered me from condemnation, the cycle of defeat.

What are some of the judgments you have made about food? When and where did those judgments begin? How does it make your heart feel when you think about guilt-free eating?

_____

_____

_____

_____

_____

_____

_____

_____

_____

_____

_____

_____

_____

_____

_____

_____

_____

_____

_____

_____

_____

_____

_____

_____

Week 9

Connie Witter

Day 25

Sin Has Lost Its Power

*"...Our old sinful selves were crucified with
Christ so that sin might lose its power in our
lives. We are no longer slaves to sin. ⁷ For
when we died with Christ we were set free
from the power of sin... ¹⁴ Sin is no longer
your master, for you no longer live under the
requirements of the law. Instead, you live
under the freedom of God's grace."*

– Romans 6:6-7, 14 NLT

Your old sinful nature died on the cross with Jesus.
Jesus gave you a brand-new nature of righteousness. By
giving you His perfect righteousness as your identity, your
failures have completely lost their power to condemn you or
define you. The law simply reminds you of how guilty you
are and how much you fail, but grace reminds you who you
are and empowers you to bear the fruit of righteousness.

Have you ever had an area of your life you felt like you
couldn't get victory over? I used to relate to the apostle
Paul when he wrote in Romans 7:18-19, 24-25: *"And I
know that nothing good lives in me, that is, in my sinful
nature. I want to do what is right, but I can't. ¹⁹ I want to
do what is good, but I don't. I don't want to do what is
wrong, but I do it anyway... ²⁴ Oh, what a miserable
person I am! Who will free me from this life that is
dominated by sin and death? ²⁵ Thank God! The answer is
in Jesus Christ our Lord..."* (NLT).

When it comes to any area in which you have struggled, including losing weight, the devil would like you to believe the lie that you have to try harder, discipline yourself more. He may have even gotten you to feel like the apostle Paul did in Romans 7, like no matter what you do, you can't make yourself eat right. You want to, but you can't. You may feel like a failure in this area, but the answer to your struggle is in coming to the throne of grace and embracing your true identity in Jesus.

Hebrews 4:15-16: *"For we do not have a high priest who is unable to empathize with our weaknesses, but we have one who has been tempted in every way, just as we are— yet he did not sin. ¹⁶ Let us then approach God's throne of grace with confidence, so that we may receive mercy and find grace to help us in our time of need"* (NIV).

Remember, Philippians 2:13 says, *"[Not in your own strength] for it is God Who is all the while effectually at work in you [energizing and creating in you the power and desire], both to will and to work for His good pleasure and satisfaction and delight"* (AMPC).

I remember the day the revelation of these Scriptures came to my heart. I had been struggling in so many areas of my life. I was trying to do right, but constantly seemed to fail.

However, when I daily began to come to God's throne of grace and ask Him to create in me the desire and power to do what pleases Him, something supernatural began to happen in me. As I began to see myself as already righteous in Jesus and looked to Him daily for the grace I needed, I saw more of the fruit of the Spirit come out in my life.

Romans 5:17 says, *"For the sin of this one man, Adam, caused death to rule over many. But even greater is God's wonderful grace and his gift of righteousness, for all who receive it will live in triumph over sin and death through this one man, Jesus Christ"* (NLT).

I have a friend who struggled with her weight her entire life. She was more than 100 pounds overweight and felt very condemned. She had tried for years to lose weight in her own strength. She would lose weight at times but would simply gain it all back. She saw herself as a failure in this area of her life.

Then she began to come to the throne of grace and believe who she is in Jesus. She began to see herself as a healthy, righteous woman in Christ. She asked Jesus daily to create in her the desire and power to exercise and to eat healthy.

We all watched as she was transformed from the inside out. She triumphed over sin and death by receiving the gift of righteousness and His overflowing grace.

Romans 6:11 says, *"...Since you are now joined with him, you must continually view yourselves as dead and unresponsive to sin's appeal while living daily for God's pleasure in union with Jesus..."* (TPT).

This verse reveals the answer to freedom! It says that since you are now one with Jesus, continually view yourself as dead to the power of sin, and continually see yourself as one with Jesus. You are one with Perfect Health! You are one with Perfect Righteousness! You are one with Perfect Love! You are defined by your oneness with Jesus!

The reason too many of God's children are still struggling in areas of their lives is because they are still defining themselves by their sin and failure. When you define yourself by the law, it will only condemn you and keep you in the vicious cycle of sin and failure. But when you continually view yourself as dead to the law of sin and death and alive as one with Jesus, you will live truly free!

Prayer: Jesus, thank You for setting me free from the power of sin. My sinful nature died with You on the cross and I am resurrected as one with You! You define my life now! I now see that my freedom is found in continually viewing myself as dead to sin's power, and continually viewing myself as one with You! You create in me the desire and power to believe who I am in You. I am not a failure! I am victorious because I am one with You!

When it comes to weight loss and eating healthy, can you relate to the apostle Paul and how he felt in Romans 7:18-19 & 24-25? How will seeing yourself as dead to sin's power and one with Jesus free you from this struggle? Talk to Jesus about the truth that was revealed to your heart in today's devotion.

_____

_____

_____

_____

_____

_____

_____

_____

_____

_____

_____

_____

_____

_____

_____

_____

_____

_____

_____

_____

_____

_____

_____

_____

_____

Day 26

Let Go of the Weight That Hinders Your Progress

"...Let us strip off every weight that slows us down, especially the sin that so easily trips us up. And let us run with endurance the race God has set before us. ² We do this by keeping our eyes on Jesus, the champion who initiates and perfects our faith."

– Hebrews 12:1-2 NLT

Hebrews chapter 11 is often referred to as the Hall of Faith. It lists men and women throughout history that dared to believe what God said about them in the face of contrary circumstances. Hebrews chapter 12 begins by referring to these men and women of faith and encourages us to strip off every weight that slows us down, especially "the sin" that trips us up. It's interesting to note that this verse doesn't say strip off "the sins," but "the sin".

The Greek word for "sin" in this verse is *harmartia* and it's actually a noun, not a verb. In other words, this verse is actually talking about stripping off the weight of your old identity. We were all sinners, defined by our sin and failure, but that's not who we are anymore. Roman 5:8-9 says that even when we were sinners, Christ died to make us righteous through our union with Him. You are a new creation! You've been given a brand-new, righteous identity in Jesus. Your sin and failure can no longer define you. Jesus defines your life now.

We've all struggled to believe what God says about us at times. Often our circumstances or failures have caused us to question:

"Is what Jesus says about me really true? Look at my life! How can I believe that there is nothing at all wrong with me?

"Jesus says I'm tall and thin like a palm tree? Look at me! Can't you see that's definitely not true about me? I lack. I can't do it. I'm a failure. I must not have enough faith."

Even as I write this, I can feel the weight of holding onto a false identity. Holding onto the weight of guilt and shame, caused by not believing what Jesus says about you, is a heavy burden to carry. Discouragement, frustration, disappointment, and feeling hopeless that your circumstances will ever change are all the result of holding onto your old identity instead of embracing your new identity in Jesus. I know that any time I'm not experiencing freedom in an area of my life, it's because I'm not believing what my good Father says about me in Christ.

So how do we strip ourselves of this weight of holding onto a false identity? How can we really believe and embrace our new identity in Jesus?

Hebrews 12:2 says, *"We do this by keeping our eyes on Jesus, the champion who initiates and perfects our faith"* (NLT).

Isn't it wonderful to know that you don't have to try hard to believe right about yourself? Not only did Jesus make you righteous, but He empowers you to believe it. He is the author and perfecter of your faith.

Galatians 2:20 says, *"My old identity has been co-crucified with Messiah and no longer lives; for the nails of his cross crucified me with him. And now the essence of this new life is no longer mine, for the Anointed One lives his life through me—we live in union as one! My new life is empowered by the faith of the Son of God who loves me so much that he gave himself for me, and dispenses his life into mine!"* (TPT).

What glorious Good News! Your old identity has been crucified with Jesus, and now Jesus lives His life through you. Your new life is empowered by the faith of Jesus, who loves you so much that He died and rose again to make you one with Him. Your new identity is defined by your union with Him! You no longer have to depend on your faith: you are empowered by His!

Ephesians 3:16-20 says, *"And I pray that he would unveil within you the unlimited riches of his glory and favor until supernatural strength floods your innermost being with his divine might and explosive power. 17 Then, by constantly using your faith, the life of Christ will be released deep inside you, and the resting place of his love will become the very source and root of your life.*

"18-19 Then you will be empowered to discover what every holy one experiences—the great magnitude of the astonishing love of Christ in all its dimensions. How deeply intimate and far-reaching is his love! How enduring and inclusive it is! Endless love beyond measurement that transcends our understanding—this extravagant love pours into you until you are filled to overflowing with the fullness of God!

"²⁰ Never doubt God's mighty power to work in you and accomplish all this. He will achieve infinitely more than your greatest request, your most unbelievable dream, and exceed your wildest imagination! He will outdo them all, for his miraculous power constantly energizes you" (TPT).

What a powerful passage of Scripture! These verses say that Jesus will unveil within you the ability to see yourself the way He sees you! As He reveals to you the unlimited riches of His view and opinion of you, supernatural strength will flood your soul with His divine might and explosive power. You'll come to know His extravagant love and be filled with the fullness of God.

Ephesians 3:20 says never doubt God's mighty power to work in you and accomplish all of this. He will achieve infinitely more than your greatest request and your most unbelievable dreams, for His miraculous power constantly energizes you. So, today, let go of that false identity and run your race of victory by keeping your eyes on Jesus. You live by His faith in you. Nothing will be impossible to you as you live as one with Him!

Prayer: Jesus, today I let go of the weight of defining myself by my old identity. I trust You to do a powerful work in me. You're the author and finisher of my faith. I'm one with You, Jesus, and I'm empowered by Your faith in me! You define who I am! Thank You for loving me into freedom!

Are you holding onto the weight of a false identity? Are there things that you have believed about yourself that have weighed you down? Are you ready to let go of the weight of defining yourself by your old identity, and turn your eyes upon Jesus, the author and finisher of your faith? Write down how today's devotion encouraged your heart.

_____

_____

_____

_____

_____

_____

_____

_____

_____

_____

_____

_____

_____

_____

_____

_____

_____

_____

_____

_____

_____

_____

_____

Day 27

Jesus—Your Way of Escape

"No temptation [regardless of its source] has overtaken or enticed you that is not common to human experience [nor is any temptation unusual or beyond human resistance]; but God is faithful [to His word—He is compassionate and trustworthy], and He will not let you be tempted beyond your ability [to resist], but along with the temptation He... will [always] provide the way out, so that you will be able to endure it [without yielding, and will overcome temptation with joy]."

– 1 Corinthians 10:13 AMP

Many years ago, I had gotten into really unhealthy eating habits. Pizza, hamburgers, french fries, and diet coke were my foods of choice. Although I didn't have a weight problem, my body was feeling the effects of my unhealthy choices. I had trained my body to like unhealthy foods and that is what it craved. French fries were often calling my name. Now, having french fries on occasion is ok, but when they become your steady diet, you know that is a problem. Our bodies need vitamins and minerals to feel strong, energetic and healthy. I wanted to be healthy, but the temptation to eat unhealthy was greater.

I had heard people say that they had asked Jesus to help them to lose weight and become healthy in their body, but they continued to struggle with overeating and unhealthy choices. So, I asked Jesus, "Why aren't You helping them? If they've asked for Your help, why are they not experiencing victory in this area of their lives?"

It wasn't until I asked Jesus to help me to make healthy choices that I discovered the answer to my question. One morning, after I had asked Jesus to help me eat healthier, I went to the grocery store. As I was checking out, I looked over at all those candy bars on the shelf and the temptation was great to buy one and eat it.

I remembered my earlier conversation with Jesus, but in that moment my flesh wanted that candy. I bought it, I ate it, and then the next thought was, *You shouldn't have eaten that. You know that doesn't make you feel good.* It was a condemning thought that was accusing me of being a failure at eating healthy.

Immediately, I turned my thoughts to Jesus and said, "Why didn't you help me overcome that temptation?" In His loving and compassionate way, He replied, "Connie, when you're tempted, I am your way of escape. I am faithful to remind you who you are, and help you make a different choice, but in that moment of temptation, you didn't ask Me to help you."

It reminded me of 1 Corinthians 10:13. Temptations come to all of us, but this verse says that God is faithful, and He won't let you be tempted beyond your ability to resist. With every temptation, He will provide a way of escape, so that you will not yield to it, but overcome it with joy. I realized in that moment why so many of God's children, including myself, fall into temptation and don't experience victory over food addictions. It's because in the moment of temptation, we don't talk to Jesus and ask Him to help us.

Because when we do, He is always faithful to send forth His Word and empower us by His Spirit to overcome every temptation with joy.

What Jesus taught me that day changed my life forever! I realized that if I really wanted to be free from my unhealthy choices and experience the healthy life my good Father desired for me, I must run to Jesus and talk to Him in the moment of my temptation. He will always provide a way of escape by creating in me the desire and power to make healthy choices and remind me that I am not a failure. I am an overcomer in Him!

As I began to talk to Jesus daily about my food choices, I found myself desiring healthy food. Jesus took the craving for diet soda completely out of my system. I haven't desired a diet coke in over 10 years. French fries no longer call my name. I truly enjoy eating salads and fruit, and I love the way they make my body feel. Jesus truly is our way of escape. He sent forth His Word to heal us and deliver us from destruction (Psalm 107:20). He is our victory over every temptation.

Jesus sent the Holy Spirit to live within you so that you could overcome every temptation. In John 14:26 Jesus said, *"...The Comforter (Counselor, Helper, Intercessor, Advocate, Strengthener, Standby), the Holy Spirit, Whom the Father will send in My name... He will teach you all things. And He will...(bring to your remembrance) everything I have told you"* (AMPC).

When you're tempted to go to food for comfort or for any other emotional reason, remember the Holy Spirit is within you. In that moment, acknowledge Him. He is your Comforter.

He will counsel you and lead you. He will strengthen you and remind you who you are in Jesus so that you can live a healthy life.

2 Timothy 1:7 says, *"For God did not give us a spirit of...fear), but [He has given us a spirit] of power and of love and of calm and well-balanced mind and discipline and self-control"* (AMPC).

You have the spirit of power, discipline and self-control. It's who you are in Jesus! You have everything you need to overcome temptation and experience victory over food addictions. So, the next time you're tempted, talk to Jesus, and agree with what He says about you. He is faithful to His Word. He is compassionate and trustworthy. He'll always provide a way of escape out of temptation and into the freedom of a healthy life.

Prayer: Jesus, in every temptation, You're my way of escape. In that moment, I will talk to You, and agree with what You say about me. I have the spirit of discipline and self-control. Food addictions have no power over me because I am one with You! Thank you, Jesus, for setting me free with Your love!

Read 1 Corinthians 10:13 again. What promise did Jesus give you in this verse? According to 2 Timothy 1:7, what is the truth about your new nature in Jesus? Write down the impact this truth had on your heart.

_____

_____

_____

_____

_____

_____

_____

_____

_____

_____

_____

_____

_____

_____

_____

_____

_____

_____

_____

_____

_____

_____

_____

_____

_____

_____

_____

_____

Week 10

Gwen Myrie & Sherry Riether

Day 28: Resurrected to a Brand-New Life—Gwen

Day 29: Only Believe—Gwen

Day 30: Deliverance from the Desert—Sherry

Day 31: Truly Free—No Going Back to Bondage—Sherry

Day 28

Resurrected to a Brand-New Life

*"Christ's resurrection is your resurrection too.
This is why we are to yearn for all that is above,
for that's where Christ sits enthroned at the place
of all power, honor, and authority!"*

– Colossians 3:1 TPT

The Resurrection of Jesus Christ is the central focus of the Gospel. It's the Good News of Christ. The apostle Paul says in Romans 1:16 that the Gospel is the power of God unto salvation! This Good News is so critical to our understanding. In the above referenced scripture, Christ's resurrection is our resurrection! When we set our hearts on this vital truth, our lives begin to transform into the very image of Christ. We are now One with Him!

1 John 4:17 states plainly, *"By living in God, love has been brought to its full expression in us so that we may fearlessly face the day of judgment, because all that Jesus now is, so are we in this world"* (TPT).

Let this powerful verse sink down deep into your heart, *"because all that Jesus now is, so are we in this world."* We are just like Jesus right now in this world. At this moment, you may be thinking that is astonishing and hard to believe because we live in this natural world and see things from an earthly perspective. That is why we need the Holy Spirit to help us see from God's perspective. The Divine Encourager was sent to help us in every area of our lives. Right now, at this moment, you are seated, enthroned at the place of all power, honor, and authority! God can't lie! He is the one who says this about you! You are resurrected to a brand-new life!

What does it mean to see things from God's perspective? In the mind of God, everything is already finished. He sees you as righteous, holy, blameless, accepted, approved, and at a healthy weight. He views you in Christ. Jesus desires that you see yourself the way He sees you.

2 Corinthians 3:18 is a powerful verse that tells us what happens to us when we see things from Jesus' perspective: *"But we all, with unveiled face, beholding as in a mirror the glory of the Lord, are being transformed into the same image from glory to glory, just as by the Spirit of the Lord"* (NKJV).

This is something that will happen to you as you exchange your glory for the glory of Jesus. The word "glory" means "the view, opinion or judgment." In the New Testament, it is always a good opinion of one resulting in praise honor and glory! [xiii] When you exchange your view, opinion, or judgments about yourself for Jesus', your life will be transformed.

Jesus wants to change the way you think about your life and body. His opinion of you will never change. His opinion of you is always good! I want to emphasize the last line of this verse, *"just as by the Spirit of the Lord."* Jesus wants to remind you that this is a work of the Holy Spirit. He only desires for you to behold him in the Word as in a mirror so you will see that as He is, so are you in this world! Glory to God! Let's look at another verse that reveals God's perspective.

2 Corinthians 5:17 says, *"Now, if anyone is enfolded into Christ, he has become an entirely new person* [creation]. *All that is related to the old order has vanished. Behold, everything is fresh and new"* (TPT, brackets added).

This is an amazing verse of scripture because it states plainly that you are a new creation. The old you died and was buried. Romans 6:4 says, *"Therefore we were buried with Him through baptism into death, that just as Christ was raised from the dead by the glory of the Father, even so we also should walk in newness of life"* (NKJV).

I am sure that by now you can see that your old man is dead. Your new identity is Christ, the Resurrected One. You no longer have to identify yourself as a failure when it comes to anything that you want to accomplish. Christ, through your union with Him, empowers you to live above because that is where He is seated. He desires for you to see your life from His amazing perspective. You're not a failure! You're more than a conqueror! You can do all things through your union with Jesus!

Now here is some more Good News! 1 Corinthians 1:30 says, *"But of Him you are in Christ Jesus, who became for us wisdom from God—and righteousness and sanctification and redemption"* (NKJV).

Let this verse be your meditation, "it is of God that you are in Christ" (1 Corinthians 1:30). Jesus is reminding you, once again, that this is His work which He does in you. Rest in the fact that you are one with the resurrected One and that you have received an abundance of grace and the free gift of righteousness. You are as you ought to be, right now. Let Jesus love the weight off of you by revealing to your heart who you really are. Sit down, and rest in His faithful love. In Christ, you are already resurrected to a brand-new life!

Prayer: Father, thank You that I no longer have to identify with the old man because when Christ died, I died. I was crucified with Him, buried with Him, and resurrected to this brand-new life! Thank You for making me a new creation and empowering me by Your Holy Spirit to be victorious in my life. I see that it is by Your Spirit, and not my efforts, that I am transformed into Your image!

How does it make your heart feel to know that you have already been resurrected to a new life? List some of the opinions that you have had of yourself and then list next to them what God says about you. Take time to ask the Holy Spirit to help you see yourself the way Jesus sees you.

_____

_____

_____

_____

_____

_____

_____

_____

_____

_____

_____

_____

_____

_____

_____

_____

_____

_____

_____

_____

_____

_____

_____

_____

_____

_____

_____

_____

Day 29

Only Believe

"While He was still speaking, some came from the ruler of the synagogue's house who said, 'Your daughter is dead. Why trouble the Teacher any further?' 36 As soon as Jesus heard the word that was spoken, He said to the ruler of the synagogue, 'Do not be afraid; only believe.'"

– Mark 5:35-36 NKJV

Something has died! Have your dreams of ever losing weight died? Have you buried your dream of ever having a healthy body? Death seems so final when you can only see things from an earthly perspective. Imagine Jairus, for a moment, his only child at the brink of death. He comes to Jesus for help and some woman with an issue of blood interrupts his miracle. He only has to get Jesus to his house, and all will be well. Jesus is talking with the woman, when messengers come from Jairus' house and say these earth-shattering and devastating words: "Your daughter is dead." Fear gripped his heart; he was powerless in its clutches! Jesus overheard the word that had been spoken and ignored it by saying to Jairus, "Do not be afraid; only believe!"

Jesus is saying the same thing to you at this very moment: only believe! Your dreams of a better life may have died. You may have held the funeral and buried them, but I am here to declare to you that Jesus said, "I am the resurrection and the life!"

It's time to lift your expectation to the One who can raise the dead and call those things that be not as though they were!

Jesus made a very powerful and thought-provoking statement to Mary in John 11:17-43. Lazarus, the brother of Mary and Martha had died. Another death! Another situation that looked hopeless! (Jesus loves to resurrect people and situations.) Jesus told Mary, "I am the resurrection and the life and even if a person dies that believes in Me, that person will live" (John 11:25).

Martha and Mary said they believed. They both believed right up to the point when Jesus said, "Roll away the stone." Then the unbelief surfaced!

"By now he stinks—he's been dead 4 days!" Then Jesus made an astounding statement to Mary, *"Did I not say to you that if you would believe you would see the glory of God?"* (John 11:40 NKJV). Wow! This is very exciting!

How long has your dream been dead and buried? How long have you struggled to lose the weight? It's hard to hold on to something that has died. If you have given up, listen again to what Jesus said, *"Did I not say to you* (dear reader) *that if you would believe, you would see the glory of God?"* Jesus is speaking to you now. Let his powerful words penetrate your heart and soul. His words give life!

I want to highlight two words: believe and glory. What does it mean to believe? Did you know that it is not your responsibility to make yourself believe? *Pisteuō* is the Greek word in this verse for "believe," and it means "to think to be true, to be persuaded of, place confidence in." [xiv]

Digging deeper to the root is *peithō*, which means "to persuade, to induce one by words to believe, to make friends of, to win one's favor, to allow one's self to be persuaded." [xv] Jesus said the Holy Spirit was sent to reveal the truth to us and to persuade us of the truth. The Holy Spirit is here to persuade you to believe what is the truth about you. Jesus said, "It is the Father in me—He does the work" (John 14:10). He brings about persuasion in our hearts.

The Greek word for "glory" is *doxa*, which means "opinion, judgment, view and in the New Testament always a good opinion concerning one, resulting in praise, honor, and glory." [xvi] God's glory is his opinion, judgement, and view. God's glory is also all that he is and all that he can do.

What does God have to say about dead things? He says, "I am the resurrection and the life!" Things cannot remain dead in the presence of Life. What is God's view of your life? Your life is hidden in God in Christ and in Him there is no condemnation, failure, hopelessness or frustration. In Him there is no death, only life! God says that you are blameless and without fault in His sight. You are more than a conqueror! You can do all things through the Christ who lives within you! God's judgement of you is that you are the righteousness of God in Christ Jesus!

Recently, I realized that I had been exalting my opinion of myself over God's opinion of me. What an eye-opening revelation. I was walking in pride because I thought I assessed my life's circumstances better than God. Imagine my shock! I never would've viewed that as pride, but it was. Anytime we view our lives through our own opinions, we are walking in pride. God gives grace to the humble, those who are willing to accept His opinion over their own (James 4:6).

Beloved, as hard as it has been for you in your struggle to lose weight, this is your time! Are you ready and willing to let go of your opinion for His? If you are, you are ready to let Jesus love that weight off of you!

Prayer: Father, thank You for encouraging me to dream again. I exchange my opinion of my life for Your opinion. You have sent your Holy Spirit to persuade my heart to believe what You say about me. Thank You for helping me rest in Your love as You persuade my heart of the truth.

What comes to your heart when you think of resurrecting your dreams of having a healthy body? Write those thoughts down and present them to Jesus. Let Him reveal the truth to your heart so that you can walk free! It's your time! Arise and shine, your light has come, God's glory is yours!

_____

_____

_____

_____

_____

_____

_____

_____

_____

_____

_____

_____

_____

_____

_____

_____

_____

_____

_____

_____

_____

_____

_____

_____

_____

_____

_____

_____

_____

Day 30

Deliverance from Wandering in the Desert

"Jesus looked at them and said, 'With man this is impossible, but not with God; all things are possible with God.'"

– Mark 10: 27 NIV

As I have been on this journey to health, the Lord has reminded me many times of the story of the Israelites in the Bible when they were delivered out of slavery to the Egyptians. Their lives were miserable in that captivity, and they cried out to God for help because they knew they could not save themselves.

God sent Moses to secure their deliverance, and off they went on their journey to freedom. The problem was, they kept going, and going, and going and it seemed like they would never arrive to their destination: The Promised Land. The promise of a life free from bondage seemed impossible to some when all they could see around them was desert.

I can imagine them saying to God, "When will we get to this free life you promised us? We used to be able to eat all we wanted and had plenty of water, but now we're stuck in this desert another day!"

When you are focused on losing weight and getting healthy, it can feel like it's taking forever, like you're not making progress and you will never hit your goal. Like you're wandering in the desert. These feelings can especially rise up when you are not seeing a change on the scale. I have experienced these feelings, and I had times when I felt like I couldn't do it for one more day.

God had provided a way for me that had brought me out of the bondage I was in. I had seen my deliverance and it was working, and yet sometimes I still experienced the feeling, "This is impossible!" I would have cravings to go back to old eating habits.

Sometimes I would fall into the trap of feeling like I was on my own in this, and start thinking thoughts like, *I used to be able to eat chips and would at least not gain any weight. Sure, I was overweight, but I didn't have to think, 'I can't eat this, or I can't eat that.'* Some days I would just yell out, "This is impossible! I just want to quit! God, you brought me out, but I can't take wandering in this desert another day!"

Then God would sweetly remind me that I was not on this journey alone. He was there strengthening me and empowering me. Just like in Isaiah 40:29, *"He gives strength to those who are tired. He gives power to those who are weak"* (NIRV). Instead of thinking of what I couldn't do, I began thinking of what God had already done in me and what He was continuing to do in my heart.

God had not left the Israelites to wander in the desert alone. He was with them, strengthening them. He provided good and nourishing food for them along the way. His plan was not, "OK, I busted you out of prison, but now you're on your own!" NO! He was on this journey with them and caring for them all the way to freedom!

The Word says, in Psalm 105:37, and 40-41, *"He brought the people of Israel out of Egypt. From among the tribes of Israel no one got tired or fell down. 40 They asked for meat, and he brought them quail. He satisfied them with manna, the bread of heaven. 41 He broke open a rock, and streams of water poured out. They flowed like a river in the desert"* (NIRV).

When God delivers you, the desert becomes an oasis! Isaiah 35:1-2 says, *"The desert and the parched land will be glad; the wilderness will rejoice and blossom. Like the crocus, 2 it will burst into bloom; it will rejoice greatly and shout for joy"* (NIV).

When I would fall into the trap of thinking I was on my own in this journey, and I would think thoughts like, *This is impossible! God I'm in the desert another day! When am I getting out of here?* God would remind me that it was His plan of deliverance for me and He didn't just "bust me out" to wander in the desert!

He was not just partially delivering me, He was completely delivering me and providing for me all along the way! You know what? I began craving healthy food! The junk food that had held me in bondage no longer was appealing to me!

There may be times when it may seem impossible to get to a healthy weight. But when you're in the presence of Jesus and Father God, you're in the very presence of doing the impossible! Remember Jesus' words in Mark 10:27, "With man this is impossible, but with God all things are possible!" He is God, and He will deliver you from wandering in the desert another day.

Prayer: Jesus, I trust Your plan of deliverance for me! You didn't give me the desire to be healthy only to leave me to figure it out on my own. You are there, You have been there, and You will be there helping me every day. When the goal seems far away, I know You are always near and You will turn my desert into a beautiful oasis!

Picture in your mind a desert land that is hot, dry, and dusty. Then picture a stream of beautiful, cool, crystal clear water flowing over the land. Suddenly, green, luscious plants start to pop up with beautiful flowers forming and blossoming. Palm trees are growing, and their leaves are gently rustling in the wind and providing shade on rich, soft grass. Isn't that inviting? This is you! God is transforming your "desert thoughts" into "life thoughts"! How does this impact your heart as you continue your journey to health?

_____

_____

_____

_____

_____

_____

_____

_____

_____

_____

_____

_____

_____

_____

_____

_____

_____

_____

_____

_____

_____

_____

Day 31

Truly Free—No Going Back to Bondage

*"Let me be clear, the Anointed one has set us free—
not partially, but completely and wonderfully free!
We must always cherish this truth and stubbornly
refuse to go back into the bondage of our past."*

– Galatians 5:1 TPT

You've started on your journey. You've left old thought patterns behind, begun eating healthier, and maybe you've even started being more active. Yet, that scale still reads the same as it did yesterday or even last week. Or perhaps the number has even gone up. This has happened to me so many times! Even during this last time when I experienced so much success, there were days, sometimes weeks, where my weight would plateau or, worse yet, I'd find I had gained weight. Those times are so frustrating and can really have an impact on your emotions and how you feel about yourself.

When you lose weight and then gain some (or all) back, it seems like you feel worse than you did before you lost the weight. Defeating and self-condemning thoughts can plague your mind. When I hit my goal weight in May of 2018, I began to eat more freely than I had been. Over a few months I found that I had put some weight back on. It felt sickening to me and the fear that I would not be able to maintain my weight loss started creeping into my mind. I actually felt fatter than I did before I lost weight! This was so ridiculous because I had in no way gained back the nearly 60 pounds I had lost. But still the self-condemning feelings came to my mind: *See! I told you so! You're not successful! You've never been successful! Who do you think you are talking about being 'Tall and slender like a palm tree?' Why should anyone listen to a word you have to say when you're obviously not in control?*

I put up with these thoughts and even entertained them for a few days. These were old familiar feelings I had before I succeeded at losing weight. I even found myself looking through my clothes to see if I had kept any of my old bigger ones, just in case I needed them.

I was feeling sorry for myself when the Holy Spirit prompted my heart and said, "Why are you giving any time to these thoughts at all? You're looking back, but that's not the direction you are going."

I thought to myself, *That's right! I don't have to listen to those thoughts anymore!*

I said, "No!" to them and stubbornly refused to go back into the bondage of my past! I began to think about the words Jesus had taught me to say over myself before I even lost one pound. "You're healthy. You're at a healthy weight. You have a healthy body. Father, You say I am perfect, and your Word says my body is Your temple (1 Corinthians 6:19). A temple cannot build itself or maintain itself. It needs a keeper and a caretaker and that is you, Father." It's the Father's job to keep and maintain it!

My heart began to leap within me!! I stopped looking for the old clothes that didn't fit me anymore and began doing a happy dance right there in my closet! I felt empowerment rise up in me again! Just as Jesus had loved the weight off of me, the Father was going to help me maintain my weight because I am His temple! What freedom there is in that! Let's read our theme verse for today again:

"Let me be clear, the Anointed one has set us free—not partially free, but completely and wonderfully free! We must always cherish this truth and stubbornly refuse to go back into the bondage of our past" (Galatians 5:1 TPT).

How do I cherish the truth? I declare my freedom in Christ! I am truly, wonderfully, completely and totally free! I stubbornly refuse to go back into the bondage of my past and own any thought that would condemn me or any thought that does not align with what God's Word says over me. These are not my thoughts anyway, because I have been set free from them! John 8:36 says, *"So if the Son sets you free, you are truly free!"* (NLT, emphasis added).

As you are walking down this path to health, I want to encourage you. You may experience moments when you feel like giving up, when it seems too much, or too hard. Those are the times to remember that you are God's temple and He's the keeper of that temple. In fact, He has already recreated you into something completely and totally new.

His Word in 2 Corinthians 5:17 says, *"Therefore, if any person is [ingrafted] in Christ (the Messiah) he is a new creation (a new creature altogether); the old [previous moral and spiritual condition] has passed away. Behold, the fresh and new has come!"* (AMPC).

You are a new creation! Not the refurbished you! Not the remodeled you! But a completely brand-new creation that never existed before! His temple. He made you and will maintain you!

Prayer: Jesus, thank You that You have truly, wonderfully, completely and totally set me free. I no longer have to live with, or even entertain, condemning thoughts that try to bring me back into the bondage of self-defeat, guilt, or shame. I am a completely new creation, the temple of God. Thank You, that You maintain Your temple!

Think about your body as the temple of God—a temple that He maintains, He cares for, and He keeps. A brand-new creation that He built! How do these truths impact your heart? Take some time today and let the Holy Spirit empower you with His encouragement. Declare your freedom today!

_____

_____

_____

_____

_____

_____

_____

_____

_____

_____

_____

_____

_____

_____

_____

_____

_____

_____

_____

_____

_____

_____

_____

_____

_____

Other Books Published by Because of Jesus Publishing

Bible Studies by Connie Witter
Because of Jesus
Living Loved, Living Free
Awake to Righteousness Volume 1
Awake to Righteousness Volume 2

Books by Connie Witter
Lies Religion Taught Me & The Truth That Set Me Free
Living Loved Living Free
P.S. God Loves You
The Inside Story Teen Devotional
The Inside Story for Girls Devotional
*Are You a Chicken Head? I Believe What Jesus
     Says!*—Children's book

Books by other Authors
Yes I Am!—Preschool Curriculum—Shannan Orr

You can purchase any of these resources at:
www.BecauseofJesus.com

We would love to hear how this book impacted your life.

To contact the authors, write to:

Because of Jesus Ministries
PO Box 3064
Broken Arrow, OK 74013-3064

Or email Because of Jesus Ministries at:

contact@becauseofjesus.com

For additional copies of this book go to:

www.becauseofjesus.com
or call 918-994-6500

References

[i] "G5485 - charis - Strong's Greek Lexicon (KJV)." Blue Letter Bible. Accessed 19 Apr, 2019. https://www.blueletterbible.org//lang/lexicon/lexicon.cfm?Strongs=G5485&t=KJV

[ii] "G3954 - parrēsia - Strong's Greek Lexicon (KJV)." Blue Letter Bible. Accessed 19 Apr, 2019. https://www.blueletterbible.org//lang/lexicon/lexicon.cfm?Strongs=G3954&t=KJV

[iii] "H7181 - qashab - Strong's Hebrew Lexicon (KJV)." Blue Letter Bible. Accessed 19 Apr, 2019. https://www.blueletterbible.org//lang/lexicon/lexicon.cfm?Strongs=H7181&t=KJV

[iv] "G2192 - echō - Strong's Greek Lexicon (KJV)." Blue Letter Bible. Accessed 19 Apr, 2019. https://www.blueletterbible.org//lang/lexicon/lexicon.cfm?Strongs=G2192&t=KJV

[v] https://www.merriam-webster.com/dictionary/struggle

[vi] "H3372 - yare' - Strong's Hebrew Lexicon (KJV)." Blue Letter Bible. Accessed 19 Apr, 2019. https://www.blueletterbible.org//lang/lexicon/lexicon.cfm?Strongs=H3372&t=KJV

[vii] https://www.merriam-webster.com/thesaurus/awe

[viii] "H6395 - palah - Strong's Hebrew Lexicon (KJV)." Blue Letter Bible. Accessed 19 Apr, 2019. https://www.blueletterbible.org//lang/lexicon/lexicon.cfm?Strongs=H6395&t=KJV

[ix] "G5485 - charis - Strong's Greek Lexicon (KJV)." Blue Letter Bible. Accessed 19 Apr, 2019. https://www.blueletterbible.org//lang/lexicon/lexicon.cfm?Strongs=G5485&t=KJV

[x] "G5463 - chairō - Strong's Greek Lexicon (KJV)." Blue Letter Bible. Accessed 19 Apr, 2019. https://www.blueletterbible.org//lang/lexicon/lexicon.cfm?Strongs=G5463&t=KJV

[xi] "G1343 - dikaiosynē - Strong's Greek Lexicon (KJV)." Blue Letter Bible. Accessed 19 Apr, 2019. https://www.blueletterbible.org//lang/lexicon/lexicon.cfm?Strongs=G1343&t=KJV

[xii] "G2919 - krinō - Strong's Greek Lexicon (KJV)." Blue Letter Bible. Accessed 19 Apr, 2019. https://www.blueletterbible.org//lang/lexicon/lexicon.cfm?Strongs=G2919&t=KJV

[xiii] "G1391 - doxa - Strong's Greek Lexicon (KJV)." Blue Letter Bible. Accessed 19 Apr, 2019. https://www.blueletterbible.org//lang/lexicon/lexicon.cfm?Strongs=G1391&t=KJV

[xiv] "G4100 - pisteuō - Strong's Greek Lexicon (KJV)." Blue Letter Bible. Accessed 19 Apr, 2019. https://www.blueletterbible.org//lang/lexicon/lexicon.cfm?Strongs=G4100&t=KJV

[xv] "G3982 - peithō - Strong's Greek Lexicon (KJV)." Blue Letter Bible. Accessed 19 Apr, 2019. https://www.blueletterbible.org//lang/lexicon/lexicon.cfm?Strongs=G3982&t=KJV

[xvi] "G1391 - doxa - Strong's Greek Lexicon (KJV)." Blue Letter Bible. Accessed 19 Apr, 2019. https://www.blueletterbible.org//lang/lexicon/lexicon.cfm?Strongs=G1391&t=KJV

Made in the USA
Monee, IL
19 November 2019